ARE YOU LOOKING FOR A SAFE, NATURAL
SUPPLEMENT TO HELP WITH:

Heart function?
Chronic Fatigue Syndrome?
Sports performance?
Weight loss?
Brain health?
Mental sharpness?
PMS?
Male infertility?

READ *THE CARNITINE CONNECTION*
TO SEE IF CARNITINE CAN WORK FOR
YOU!

St. Martin's Paperbacks Titles
by Winifred Conkling

THE
CARNITINE
CONNECTION

WINIFRED CONKLING

A Lynn Sonberg Book

St. Martin's Paperbacks

THE CARNITINE CONNECTION

Copyright © 2000 by Lynn Sonberg Book Associates.

ISBN: 0-312-97458-2

Printed in the United States of America

St. Martin's Paperbacks edition/ April 2000

10 9 8 7 6 5 4 3 2 1

Contents

Author's Note

THIS BOOK IS FOR INFORMATIONAL PURPOSES only. It is not intended to take the place of medical advice from a trained medical professional. Readers are advised to consult a physician or other qualified health professional regarding treatment of all of their health problems or before acting on any of the information in this book.

Research on carnitine is ongoing and subject to conflicting interpretations. As a result, there is no guarantee that what we know about carnitine will not change with time.

Foreword

KENNETH SINGLETON, M.D.

IN MY MEDICAL PRACTICE, I ENCOUNTER A LOT OF tired and weary people. Many drag themselves into my office complaining that they find it difficult to make it through the day without collapsing in exhaustion. Exercise and even daily routines that their bodies once handled with ease have become insurmountable challenges. They feel bone-tired all the time, from the time the alarm clock sounds in the morning to the time they set the alarm that evening.

After ruling out possible medical problems, I often find myself designing strategies to help my patients handle their debilitating fatigue. While a number of natural remedies and lifestyle changes can help to manage fatigue, I have found the vitaminlike substance carnitine to be one of the most useful "antifatigue" treatments available, especially when it is combined with the nutrient coenzyme Q10, or CoQ10. Patients who use carnitine often report that they have rediscovered their youthful vigor and feel years younger after taking the supplement. In many cases, the results are nothing less than miraculous.

Carnitine does much more than energize the weary. It also helps improve muscle performance by fueling the energy factories in the cells. As you might suspect, this can be a real asset to athletes who want to enhance their physical performance. In my practice I often encounter amateur and professional athletes, especially bodybuilders, who tell me that they want to use hormones and creatine and other supplements to enhance their performance. They don't want to hear about the possible side effects; they want results. Instead of using the supplements they suggest, I urge them to use carnitine, which I consider to be safer and every bit as effective as other ergogenic aids.

While the energizing effects of carnitine are impressive, the supplement can do much more. I consistently recommended carnitine to two other groups of patients: those who are trying to lose weight and those who are fighting cardiovascular disease. Carnitine helps the body burn fat more efficiently, making it an excellent supplement for people who need to shed unwanted pounds. It also helps lower blood fats, especially triglycerides, and when combined with vitamin C it strengthens the blood vessels. Because of these benefits, I routinely prescribe carnitine to most of my patients who are at risk for cardiovascular disease. For those people who have already developed heart disease, particularly congestive heart failure, carnitine is essential. I continue to be amazed at how effective carnitine is for treating heart failure in people who are resistant to even the best conventional treatments.

Despite its many benefits, one of the problems with supplements like carnitine is that people don't know how they work or how they can be used safely and effectively. *The Carnitine Connection* provides readers with a simple explanation of what this extremely useful nutrient can do in many situations, both for people who are healthy and for those with health problems. This book is an excellent resource for people who are interested in strengthening their hearts, improving their physical and mental performance, increasing their energy, or simply maintaining their current state of good health. In my opinion, carnitine is one supplement that belongs in virtually everyone's medicine cabinet, and *The Carnitine Connection* is one book that belongs on virtually everyone's book shelf.

—Kenneth Singleton, M.D., M.P.H.

Introduction

FROM THE MOMENT OF CONCEPTION TO THE MO-
ment of death, our cells create and burn energy.
Specifically, we rely on the cell's mitochondria—
the so-called powerhouses of the cell—to work
tirelessly to convert nutrients into energy. When
the mitochondria's energy system works as it
should, we feel like the Energizer Bunny. When
the mitochondria grow weary or work less efficiently, our bodies slow down and we feel as if
our batteries need to be recharged.

So, how can you keep your mitochondria
functioning at peak capacity? One way is to consume all the nutrients you need to keep the
body's energy-production system working its
best. One of the essential nutrients for energy
production is the vitaminlike compound known
as carnitine. Carnitine works by fueling cells' mitochondria. Specifically, it increases the metabolism of long-chain fatty acids. To produce
energy, the mitochondria need to have access to
certain nutrients needed for metabolism, including carnitine.

This simple nutritional supplement can have
a profound influence on your energy level,
weight, cardiovascular function, mental health,
and overall health. In fact, its impressive performance in treating a wide range of health problems has made carnitine—"the energy vitamin"—

one of the hottest new supplements available in health food stores today.

It would be difficult to overestimate the importance of carnitine to your physical and mental health. Carnitine exists in almost every cell of the body, and it plays a crucial role in your overall health. Low levels of carnitine have been linked to fatigue, weakness, cardiovascular disease, and mental decline, among other health problems.

Many of the health problems triggered by carnitine insufficiency are treated using prescription drugs, which tend to be expensive and often have adverse side effects. In many cases, people can address their health problems naturally, without turning to prescription drugs. The secret, of course, is taking supplemental carnitine.

This book explains how carnitine works in the body and how it can work for you. Consider all that carnitine can do for you:

- Carnitine boosts the cells' energy-production system, especially when taken in combination with coenzyme Q10. Carnitine naturally increases energy, without the harmful side effects associated with nervous system stimulants.
- Carnitine enhances sports performance and endurance while reducing the tissue damage that can occur during exercise.
- Carnitine helps you lose weight by boosting the energy production of the cells.

- Carnitine helps keep triglyceride levels low and "good" HDL cholesterol levels high, thus helping to prevent heart disease.
- Carnitine helps prevent cardiac arrhythmia, the cause of approximately one-third of all heart attack deaths.
- Acetyl-L-carnitine, a form of carnitine, increases mental energy, relieves depression, and helps prevent Alzheimer's disease.
- Carnitine enhances the immune system, helping the body resist illness.
- Carnitine also has been shown to be effective in the treatment of a number of other health problems, ranging from male infertility, to diabetes, to tissue healing following surgery.

In addition to describing the many benefits of carnitine supplementation, *The Carnitine Connection* also provides information from experts on how the substance can be used safely and effectively to treat many health problems. Of course, the information presented here is not intended to take the place of consultation with a trained medical professional. Always consult your doctor before using carnitine in the management of a health problem. Carnitine can be an excellent addition to your health regimen, but your primary physician should oversee your total treatment plan.

ONE

What Is Carnitine?

CARNITINE MAY NOT ENJOY THE POPULAR ACclaim of other nutritional supplements, but it deserves recognition and appreciation for its essential role in the healthy functioning of the body. Every form of life—from the simplest single-cell organism to the unfathomably complex human body—depends on carnitine for energy production within the cells. Without carnitine, life would not exist in the form that we know it.

Carnitine is essential for energy production and it is found in almost every cell in our bodies. It is present in greatest concentrations in the heart, brain, muscles, and testicles, all of which require the generation of intensive concentrations of energy.

At the most basic level, carnitine shuttles fat (or long-chain fatty acids, to be more precise) into the energy centers or mitochondria of the cells, where the fat can be burned to produce energy. Without enough carnitine, the cell's furnace cannot work at peak efficiency and the cell's energy-production system slows down or stalls. When the body has sufficient carnitine reserves, the cells can burn more fat and generate more energy.

In addition to generating energy, fat burning creates a number of other health benefits. For example, carnitine-enhanced fat burning prevents the accumulation of excess fat in the heart, liver, and muscles; if allowed to build up, this fat can contribute to a number of different health problems, such as diabetes, heart disease, and high triglyceride levels. And, of course, fat that is converted to energy is not stored in the body in the form of excess pounds.

Carnitine helps with weight loss because it allows and encourages the body to burn fat stores and convert them to energy. When carnitine levels dwindle, the mitochondria burn less fat for energy, leaving a person feeling wiped out and susceptible to weight gain. Fat not burned by the mitochondria accumulates in the body tissues. Ultimately, low levels of carnitine can cause both weight gain and a decrease in physical and mental energy.

Because of the essential link between carnitine and energy production, carnitine supplementation holds special promise for athletes eager to improve their physical endurance and sports performance. A number of studies show that carnitine can enhance aerobic performance, allowing athletes to exercise longer without fatigue. In one study, well-trained runners who took 2 grams of carnitine per day in divided dosages increased their maximum running speed by a remarkable 5.7 percent. Keep in mind that these well-conditioned athletes were already performing near their optimal levels; less well-trained athletes may notice even more significant improvements in their performance. All athletes need to have a sufficient amount of carnitine in their cells to optimize performance.

Not Quite a Vitamin, Not Quite an Amino Acid

Carnitine is often referred to as "the energy vitamin," but it is not really a vitamin at all. Strictly speaking, a vitamin is a substance that cannot be produced by the body and must be obtained through food. Because the body can synthesize carnitine from the amino acids lysine and methionine, carnitine is not a true vitamin.

Some people classify carnitine as an amino acid, but it is not a true amino acid either. While carnitine has a chemical structure similar to many amino acids, technically it is a nitrogen-containing, short-chain carboxylic acid. Confused? In simple terms, carnitine is a water-soluble, vitaminlike compound similar to the B-complex group of vitamins.

Carnitine can be produced by the body or obtained through food. As the parents of healthy young children know, most youngsters have a seemingly endless supply of energy. One of the reasons for this bountiful reserve of energy is that children's bodies tend to be replete with carnitine, provided they eat a well-balanced diet. Unfortunately, the amount of carnitine produced by the body declines with age; by the time a person reaches his 30s or 40s, his carnitine reserves begin to become depleted and that all-too-familiar feeling of fatigue begins to set in. But there is hope: Taking a daily dose of supplemental carnitine may be sufficient to boost carnitine levels back to their youthful levels.

Types of Carnitine

Carnitine is sold in two main forms: L-carnitine and acetyl-L-carnitine. Both forms can be used by the body. In fact, L-carnitine breaks down into acetyl-L-carnitine when it is converted into energy.

Both substances have healing effects. Generally speaking, L-carnitine is most effective at healing the heart; acetyl-L-carnitine is best at enhancing metabolism in the brain. Both forms are useful in encouraging weight loss and boosting overall energy.

A Brief Primer on Carnitine

Researchers first identified carnitine nearly 100 years ago, but they had no idea what the strange substance was or what it did in the body. In 1905 scientists in Russia and Germany isolated carnitine from the muscle tissue of several animals. They named the substance carnitine, using the Latin root *carn*, meaning flesh or meat.

More than 40 years passed before scientists realized that carnitine was essential for growth and development. In the 1950s, researchers began to appreciate the critical role that carnitine plays in energy production, but they did not yet understand the magnitude of its importance. In fact, it was not until the 1970s that scientists identified the first diseases associated with carnitine deficiency; only then did carnitine first begin to receive the respect it deserved.

Once researchers focused on the role of carnitine and energy, they recognized that people who suffered from severe carnitine deficiency also experienced life-threatening symptoms, such as heart failure and muscle loss. What, they wondered, was the link between muscle tissue and this mysterious substance, carnitine?

Over time, researchers began to put the pieces of the puzzle together, linking carnitine to energy production within the cells. They now know that carnitine levels naturally decline with age, causing a growing feeling of fatigue that often accompanies aging. The gradual depletion of carnitine levels rarely causes dramatic, diagnosable symptoms of carnitine deficiency. Instead, the steady decline causes a gradual erosion of energy, which can be more insidious and more difficult to identify as a consequence of carnitine deficiency.

In simple terms, when the cells of the body don't have enough carnitine to keep their mitochondria fueled with energy-producing fat, the cells become progressively weaker. This weakness eventually causes other medical problems. Many experts believe, for example, that low levels of carnitine may contribute to a number of serious illnesses associated with aging, including heart disease, Alzheimer's disease, and cancer. Some researchers even see carnitine deficiency and damage to the mitochondria as one of the leading causes of aging itself.

What causes carnitine levels to decline? Several factors seem to contribute to the problem:

- *Many Americans aren't consuming enough carnitine in their daily diets*. In attempting to promote good health, many people eschew carnitine-rich foods, such as red meat and dairy products, because these foods tend to contain high levels of unhealthful saturated fats. By rejecting foods rich in carnitine, these people eliminate a major source of this important nutrient.

• *Americans need to exercise more in order to encourage the use of carnitine by the body.* Exercise increases the body's synthesis of carnitine; a sedentary lifestyle can contribute to low levels of carnitine, which, in turn, can contribute to feelings of fatigue. When fatigue sets in, many people find it still more difficult to find the energy to exercise. Countless studies have documented the numerous benefits associated with exercise. (Some of the benefits of exercise are described in Chapter 9.) The improved synthesis of carnitine is yet another reason to get moving.

• *The body may use up its carnitine reserves in the battle against toxic exposures.* Exposure to environmental toxins may contribute to carnitine deficiency. In such cases, the carnitine used to clear toxins from the body cannot be used in the production of energy. The more pollutants the body encounters, the greater the body's demand for carnitine for both energy production and toxic cleanup. The greater your individual exposure to environmental toxins, the greater your need for supplemental carnitine.

Taken together, these factors help to explain why we tend to experience both an energy shortage and a carnitine shortage as we grow older. Once again, these deficiencies can be overcome with simple carnitine supplementation as described in Chapter 9.

Carnitine in the Body

While most Americans don't know much about carnitine and how it works, scientists have spent several decades studying this nutrient. Thousands of studies have found carnitine to be both safe and highly effective in the treatment of a number of medical problems. For example, for more than 20 years, doctors have prescribed carnitine and CoQ10 (both separately and together) to treat heart disease, stroke, diabetes, and other ailments.

Many of the studies explored the role of carnitine in early childhood development. Human beings need a reliable supply of carnitine from our earliest days in the womb to our final moments of life. Because fetuses obtain carnitine from their mothers, carnitine levels can drop in women during pregnancy. During the first six months of life, infants cannot produce a sufficient supply of carnitine; they must obtain carnitine from breast milk, cow milk–based formula, or carnitine-enriched soy formula.

Without enough carnitine, a child's growth and development may be stunted. These carnitine-deficient children may develop muscle weakness, heart disorders, excessive fatigue, learning disabilities, and countless other life-threatening problems. Although carnitine deficiency is relatively rare in children, approximately 375,000 infants are born each year with one of several medical disorders that interfere with the body's ability to produce carnitine. For these children, doctors prescribe carnitine supplements, sold under the brand name Carnitor; carnitine is one of a few nutritional supplements that is sold as a prescription medicine as well as an over-the-counter supplement.

What makes carnitine so important to the human body? To appreciate this simple nutrient, you must understand the many essential roles it plays in the body.

- *Carnitine stokes the energy-producing furnaces of the cells.* Carnitine literally moves fatty acids (the fuel) across the membrane of the energy-producing organs in the cells known as mitochondria (the furnace) where the fat can be converted into energy. Carnitine is absolutely essential for energy production; your body could have all the fuel (fat) it needs, but without carnitine to transfer it into the mitochondria, the system breaks down and energy isn't produced.
- *Carnitine keeps the mitochondria cleared of the waste products caused by energy production.*

Carnitine also transfers out of the cells the waste generated by burning fatty acids. If the body lacks enough carnitine to keep the mitochondria furnaces clean, energy production will suffer and toxins will collect in the mitochondria. Over time, these toxins can damage the DNA in the mitochondria, which can alter the function of the cell. When the mitochondria are damaged, they can no longer contribute to energy production.

- *Carnitine plays an essential role in the production of hormones.* Carnitine is required in the chemical production of many hormones, which, in turn, orchestrate a number of functions within the body. Carnitine deficiency can create hormonal havoc in the body.

- *Carnitine helps prevent the buildup of excessive fat reserves.* Carnitine helps the body maintain healthy levels of triglycerides and cholesterol. High levels of these blood lipids (or fats) contribute to heart disease and stroke. Carnitine also helps prevent the buildup of fat in the tissues, which causes obesity and a wide range of weight-related health problems.

- *Carnitine helps prevent dangerous blood clots, including those that cause stroke or heart attack.* Carnitine prevents the red blood cells from clumping together to form clots. Blood clots can block the arteries, restricting blood flow to the heart (causing a heart attack) or to the brain (causing a stroke).

- *Carnitine strengthens the cell membranes.* Strong membranes keep cells functioning at peak capacity and protect against viral infections. Weak cell walls can cause a number of health problems.
- *Carnitine assists in the production of red blood cells.* Carnitine is necessary for the production of porphyrin, which is needed to make red blood cells.

Where Does Carnitine Come From?

The body can get carnitine in one of three ways:

- **Your body can make it.** Carnitine can be synthesized in relatively small amounts from the amino acids lysine and methionine. To do so, however, the liver needs sufficient amounts of vitamin C, vitamin B_6 niacin, thiamin, and iron. (A deficiency in any of these nutrients can halt the production of carnitine in the body.) Typically, our bodies use amino acids to produce about 25 percent of the carnitine we need; the rest must be obtained through food or supplements.

- **You can consume carnitine in your daily diet.** The average person consumes between 50 and 200 milligrams of carnitine per day as part of the daily diet. The best sources of carnitine include meat (beef, sheep, lamb) and dairy products; it is also found in avocados. As a general rule, though, plant-based foods contain very little carnitine. Clearly, it is essential that people consume a diet containing sufficient amounts of essential amino acids in order to allow the body to produce sufficient amounts of carnitine.

- **You can take carnitine supplements.** Supplemental carnitine can be helpful in obtaining sufficient levels of this important nutrient. Vegetarians in particular should consider carnitine supplementation since many of them eat neither meat nor dairy products. Many experts believe that virtually everyone could benefit from carnitine supplementation from age 40, because the body produces less carnitine as it ages.

It can be difficult to know if you are getting enough carnitine through your daily diet. Symptoms of possible carnitine deficiency include confusion, heart pain, weak muscles, and obesity.

As this brief description of the role of carnitine in the body shows, carnitine performs essential functions in the body. Optimal amounts of carnitine are needed to achieve optimal health. While carnitine taken alone provides important health benefits, researchers have found that carnitine supplements can be made still more effective when combined with the antioxidant CoQ10. Chapter 2 describes in detail the synergy between carnitine and CoQ10.

TWO

The One-Two Punch: Carnitine and CoQ10

CARNITINE OFFERS INCREDIBLE HEALTH BENEFITS when taken alone—and researchers now recognize that those benefits can be reinforced and strengthened when carnitine is taken in combination with a second supplement known as coenzyme Q10. There are 10 types of CoQ; CoQ10 is the most active form for humans.

The body uses both carnitine and CoQ10 in the production of energy at the cellular level. A coenzyme is a chemical that works with an enzyme to complete a chemical reaction. While carnitine helps to transport fatty acids into the mitochondria of the cells, where they can be converted into energy, CoQ10 actually helps in the chemical reaction that causes the production of energy within the cell. An inadequate supply of either carnitine or CoQ10 can thwart energy production and compromise overall health.

For more than two decades, researchers and doctors in Europe and Japan have recommended the combination of carnitine and CoQ10 to their patients. Studies have repeatedly shown that the two supplements work together safely and effectively, with no known negative side effects. In recent years, physicians in the United States have begun to appreciate the value of these supplements, especially when used together.

Appreciating CoQ10

CoQ10 is a fascinating molecule that can be produced by every cell in the body. Because of its ubiquitous presence in the body, it is sometimes referred to as ubiquinone. Like carnitine, CoQ10 can be synthesized by the body or consumed in the daily diet.

The body can make its own CoQ10 by performing a chemical reaction using the amino acid tyrosine, eight vitamins, and several trace minerals. Because this process of CoQ10 synthesis involves a number of ingredients, it can break down if your body is lacking any of the required vitamins or minerals in sufficient quantities. Many people do not have enough of all the key ingredients to allow the body to produce enough CoQ10 to meet all of its physical demands.

Likewise, most people do not obtain enough CoQ10 through the foods they eat. CoQ10 is found in certain foods, most notably organ meats, oily fish (which also contain EPA, eicosapentaenoic acid), and whole grains. For most people, the recommended dose of CoQ10 is 60 to 90 milligrams (mg) a day. It can be quite difficult for the average person to consume 90 mg CoQ10 through diet alone. There is an easier way: Supplements of CoQ10 can provide this necessary nutrient at optimal levels to meet the body's physical demands. Natural levels of both carnitine and CoQ10 decline with age, so supplementation may be essential for optimal health.

When taken together, carnitine and CoQ10 help to maintain a youthful level of energy and health. Together they keep the powerhouses of the cells—the mitochondria—working efficiently. In effect, the one-two punch of carnitine and CoQ10 provide a virtual Fountain of Youth for the cells. These supplements can reinforce and rejuvenate the body's energy system, leaving you feeling more energetic and younger than you have felt in years.

There may be more at stake than feeling peppy and walking with an extra spring in your step. A number of studies have found that as cells age and become deficient in CoQ10, the body becomes more susceptible to cancer, heart disease, Parkinson's disease, and other health problems. Some researchers believe that deficiencies in carnitine and CoQ10 may be partially responsible for the increase in cardiovascular disease and cancer that tends to accompany aging.

Fortunately, you may be able to reverse the negative health consequences associated with deficiencies of carnitine and CoQ10. By taking supplemental carnitine and CoQ10, you may be able to keep the mitochondria within your cells healthy and well supplied with nutrients.

The History of CoQ10

Researchers did not discover CoQ10 until 1953, when Dr. Frederick Crane, the so-called Father of CoQ10 research, located a strange substance in the mitochondria of cauliflower. Crane, a plant physiologist at the University of Wisconsin, initially assumed that the substance was somehow related to the A vitamins, but later observations made him realize the substance was something altogether different. He continued to conduct research on the substance and later found it in the mitochondria of beef heart.

By the late 1950s, other researchers began to ask questions about CoQ10. In 1958 biochemist Karl Folkers of the Institute for Biomedical Research at the University of Texas at Austin and researchers at a pharmaceutical company identified the chemical structure of CoQ10 and soon developed a way to synthesize it. At the time, the scientists did not appreciate the significance of their discovery. Since CoQ10 was a natural substance, it could not be patented, and it was expensive to produce. The pharmaceutical company sold the technology for the production of CoQ10 to Japanese researchers. Their modifications led to a more economical fermentation process for the production of CoQ10.

While this technology was being developed, Dr. Crane continued his research into the role of CoQ10 in the cells. He found that CoQ10 was found not simply in the mitochondria but throughout each cell. Although both Drs. Crane and Folkers were dedicated to research on CoQ10, at the time most other American scientists failed to recognize the importance of the substance.

During the late 1950s and 1960s, Japanese researchers experimented with CoQ10 and its role in the body. They soon discovered that CoQ10 was effective in the treatment of congestive heart failure, a condition that does not respond well to most traditional treatments. Today, more than 6 million Japanese take CoQ10 for the treatment of heart disease. Western researchers paid little attention to this CoQ10 breakthrough; they believed the most significant changes in heart disease would involve open heart surgery and other surgical solutions rather than a simple nutritional supplement.

During this period, researchers also recognized for the first time that CoQ10 also was a powerful antioxidant. Antioxidants help the body neutralize free radicals in the cells. Free radical damage has been found to contribute to a range of diseases and medical problems, including cancer, heart disease, Alzheimer's disease, arthritis, and other problems associated with aging. Free radicals are one of the metabolic by-products of energy production in the cell; CoQ10 appears to protect the cells and the mitochondria by cleaning up these free radicals before they can damage the cells.

Now, even Western researchers appreciate the probable importance of CoQ10 in both energy production and the health of the cells. Even those scientists who once dismissed CoQ10 as a substance of little importance now wondered whether it did in fact play a crucial role in the body. Research on CoQ10 soon began in earnest.

Research on CoQ10

Studies have found that CoQ10 can protect and strengthen the heart, protect the brain, and revitalize the body's immune system. Consider the evidence.

CoQ10 and the Heart

Some of the most impressive studies done on CoQ10 involve the role of the supplement in the treatment of cardiovascular disease. The Japa-

nese began using CoQ10 to treat heart disease in
the 1960s; interest in the United States began in
1972, when researchers found that people with
heart disease tend to be severely deficient in
CoQ10. Subsequent research done by Dr. Folkers's and his colleagues found CoQ10 deficiency
in a majority of people with heart disease.
Through heart tissue biopsies, a CoQ10 deficiency was found in 50 to 75 percent of patients
with various types of heart disease, according to
Dr. Folkers's work published in the *Proceedings
of the National Academy of Sciences of the United
States of America* in 1985. Clinical studies were
begun to find out whether taking supplemental
CoQ10 could help to prevent or reverse heart
disease. Since the 1970s, more than 50 studies
have demonstrated the effectiveness of CoQ10 in
the treatment of people with heart disease.

One of the most impressive studies was conducted between 1985 and 1993 by Dr. Folkers
and Dr. Peter Langsjoen, a cardiologist in Tyler,
Texas. The study involved 424 people with several types of heart disease; they were treated
with both CoQ10 and conventional medicine. To
assess their progress, the study participants were
evaluated according to the New York Heart Association functional scale, which rates heart disease from I (the least serious) to IV (the most
serious).

After taking CoQ10, fully 58 percent of the
study participants improved by one category, 28

percent moved up two categories, and 1.2 percent moved up three categories. In addition, 43 percent of the study participants improved to the point that they could cut back or eliminate some of their cardiac medications. Many medications used to treat cardiovascular disease can have unpleasant side effects, including fatigue, nausea, and dizziness. CoQ10 offers other health benefits by allowing a patient to limit or eliminate dependence on those cardiac medications that have harmful side effects. CoQ10, like carnitine, has no known harmful side effects.

Congestive Heart Failure. Many patients with heart failure can benefit from supplemental CoQ10. When the heart has been damaged and can no longer pump efficiently but has not failed outright, a person is said to be suffering from congestive heart failure. When this occurs, the kidneys respond to the reduced blood circulation by retaining salt and water in the body, which adds additional stress to the heart and makes matters worse.

Congestive heart failure can affect either the right or left side of the heart. The left side pumps oxygen-rich blood from the lungs to the rest of the body. The right side of the heart pumps the oxygen-depleted blood back from the body to the lungs, where the oxygen is replenished. When the left side of the heart is damaged, the blood backs up into the lungs, causing wheezing and shortness of breath (even during rest), fatigue, sleep disturbances, and a dry, hacking, nonproductive cough when lying down. When the right side of the heart is damaged, the blood collects in the legs and liver, causing swollen feet and ankles, swollen neck veins, pain below the ribs, fatigue, and lethargy. People with congestive heart failure tend to have abnormally low levels of CoQ10; they also have many problems or abnormalities with the mitochondria of their cells, probably caused by the low levels of healing CoQ10.

CoQ10 is especially important in the treatment of congestive heart failure, a disease that often is fatal. While some traditional medications can improve heart function temporarily, they often delay death by no more than a few months or years at best. The five-year survival rate for people with congestive heart failure is 50 percent, and many people with the condition suffer from severe functional disabilities.

CoQ10 offers hope in treating congestive heart failure by actually changing how the heart functions and by strengthening the cells. Unfortunately, many physicians are more accustomed to managing the symptoms of disease than in using nutritional supplements to reverse the situation.

Many researchers recommend that their patients begin taking CoQ10 supplements long before the symptoms of heart failure set in. Since levels of CoQ10 begin to drop off in midlife, it

makes sense to consider taking CoQ10 supplements by the time you reach your 40th birthday.
Of course, there's no reason not to start after 40,
but the sooner you use CoQ10, the greater your
chance of avoiding problems associated with
CoQ10 deficiency. By keeping levels of CoQ10 at
youthful levels, you may be able to improve
heart function and protect your mitochondria.

Angina Pectoris. Some 3 million Americans suffer from angina, a painful attack that occurs
when the heart muscle does not get enough oxygen. (This is known as *myocardial ischemia*.)
Most angina attacks occur when the heart, damaged by high blood pressure and coronary artery
disease, is stressed by physical exertion, emotional upset, excessive excitement, or even digestion of a heavy meal. Attacks can be brought on
by walking outside on a cold day, jogging to
catch a bus, or hearing particularly distressing
news. Angina attacks often serve as painful re-
minders that the heart has been damaged, and a
full-blown heart attack may follow unless steps
are taken to mend your ailing heart.

CoQ10 can help in the treatment of angina
pectoris. As part of a double-blind study, (one in
which neither the doctor nor the patient knew
who was to receive medication and who would
receive a placebo, or "dummy pill") 12 people
with angina pectoris were give 150 mg CoQ10
daily for four weeks. When compared with the

study participants receiving a placebo (dummy pill), those taking CoQ10 experienced a 53 percent reduction in the frequency of their angina attacks. In addition, those people taking CoQ10 were able to significantly increase the amount of time they could exercise on a treadmill.

Recovery from Heart Surgery. Researchers also have had impressive results in using CoQ10 during recovery from heart surgery. This finding was demonstrated by a series of fascinating Australian studies on heart function. In the first study, the researchers sacrificed a group of young and old rats; their hearts were placed in a device that kept them beating artificially. The researchers then placed the hearts under excessive stress; a rat's heart typically beats 300 times per minute, but the stress test involved accelerating the heart rate to more than 500 beats per minute for two hours. At the end of the test, the young hearts were able to recover 45 percent of their initial function, while the old hearts recovered only 17 percent of their function.

During the second phase, one group of rats was given CoQ10 for six weeks, while the other group was given a placebo. The rats were sacrificed and the heartbeat marathon was duplicated. The young rat hearts performed the same, whether they had received CoQ10 earlier or not. The old hearts treated earlier with CoQ10, on the other hand, recovered at the same rate as the

young hearts. In other words, the hearts of old
rats that had been given CoQ10 performed just
as well as the hearts of young rats.

What impact could this finding have on the
treatment of human hearts? Researchers know
that older people (those over age 70) tend to
have more trouble recovering from heart surgery
than younger people (those under age 60). Researchers believe that the problem stems from
what is known as reperfusion injury. During
heart surgery, the heart is deprived of oxygen
and blood, just as it is during a heart attack.
When the circulation is restarted, the body experiences a rush of oxygen that causes extreme
free radical damage to the heart tissue. Free radicals are unstable cells that tend to "steal" electrons from neighboring cells. Could CoQ10 help
to neutralize these free radicals and prevent
damage to the heart caused by surgery?

To test the theory, cardiologists experimented
with small pieces of human heart tissue that had
been removed during surgery. They bathed the
heart tissue in a solution that provided it with
oxygen and glucose, and ran an electric current
through the solution to cause the heart tissue to
"beat." Researchers then measured the strength
of the heart muscle contractions.

As part of the experiment, the tissue was deprived of oxygen and glucose for an hour to sim-
ulate the experience of open heart surgery. Then
the oxygen and glucose was restored, causing

free radicals to be released. In this situation, the younger heart muscles recovered 70 percent of their strength (based on the intensity of the contractions), while the older heart muscles regained just 49 percent of their strength.

To test the impact of CoQ10 on the heart, the researchers administered CoQ10 to the heart tissue for 30 minutes before repeating the oxygen- and glucose-deprivation experiment. As in the rat heart experiment, the young hearts did not respond differently when pretreated with CoQ10, while the old hearts showed marked improvement. In fact, old heart tissue pretreated with CoQ10 actually recovered an astounding 72 percent of its contraction strength, slightly better than the recovery rate of the young hearts.

One should not conclude from this experiment that CoQ10 is effective only in older hearts. Researchers suspect that CoQ10 helps fight against heart disease at any age because it is such an effective antioxidant. CoQ10 can help prevent free radicals from damaging the heart in the first place. Studies also suggest that CoQ10 can help block the formation of cholesterol in the body, which also minimizes the risk of developing heart disease.

As discussed in Chapter 6, the combination of carnitine and CoQ10 offers even more dramatic benefits. Together, carnitine and CoQ10 help the body maintain healthy levels of cholesterol and other body lipids. Carnitine lowers triglyceride levels and raises HDL (the protective form of cholesterol), while CoQ10 lowers overall cholesterol levels. For more information on carnitine heart health, see Chapter 6.

CoQ10 and the Brain

Recent research has focused on the effect of CoQ10 on degenerative neurological diseases, such as Huntington's disease and Lou Gehrig's disease (also known as *amyotrophic lateral sclerosis*, or ALS). For the most part, doctors can offer little hope to people suffering from these conditions, but CoQ10 may hold some promise for healing.

Research done at Massachusetts General Hospital in Boston looked at the role of CoQ10 in preventing neurological disorders. First, researchers administered a brain poison to older animals, in order to bring on a physical state similar to that caused by Huntington's disease or ALS in humans. Those animals that had been taking supplemental CoQ10 experienced much less damage caused by the poison, compared with the animals that did not receive the CoQ10. Clinical trials on humans are under way to examine whether CoQ10 can help to prevent or stall the course of these illnesses in people.

CoQ10 and the Immune System

A number of studies have shown that both carnitine and CoQ10 help to strengthen the immune response, especially in people with compromised immune systems. On a strictly anecdotal level, people taking supplemental CoQ10 often report that they have not had a cold since they began taking it.

But how does CoQ10 work its magic on immunity? The jury is still out, but there are several theories. Some researchers speculate that because CoQ10 is an antioxidant, it may directly protect the immune cells from damage caused by free radicals. Others believe that CoQ10 (as well as other antioxidants) may regulate the genes that control cell activity. Still other researchers believe that one of the reasons the immune system falters as we age is that the cells themselves communicate less effectively; CoQ10, they argue, may help to facilitate communication among the immune-system cells, allowing them to offer a timely and powerful response to any potential threat.

Research done in the 1990s indicates that CoQ10 may help to fight cancer by strengthening the immune system. In 1991 researchers found that some people suffering from cancer had lower levels of CoQ10 in their blood than people without cancer. Additional research has found that CoQ10 makes immune cells known as T-cells more efficient; T-cells are helpful in searching for and destroying cancer cells in the body.

*   *   *

As stated earlier, CoQ10 taken in combination with carnitine makes the benefits of carnitine still more dramatic. Chapter 3 describes how carnitine and CoQ10 work together to support the body's energy production system.

THREE

No More Fatigue: Carnitine and Optimal Energy

CARNITINE HAS EARNED A REPUTATION AS THE "energy vitamin" for good reason. This simple supplement can have a profound effect on energy production within the cells, taking you from fatigued and exhausted to feeling fantastic and energetic. Carnitine can rejuvenate your energy system by fortifying the mitochondria of the cells, the structures in the cells that are responsible for energy production. By keeping your body supplied with optimal amounts of carnitine, you can achieve optimal energy levels.

By age 40, carnitine levels tend to taper off, and energy levels begin to decline. At this age, many people begin to feel a bit weary and middle aged. With a full supply of carnitine, you may be able to reverse the energy decline associated with aging. Not only will you feel better, but your body also will have more energy to fight off infections and diseases that tend to plague people later in life.

NOTE: If you are experiencing a significant problem with fatigue, you should consult your doctor to rule out the possibility that you suffer from a thyroid dysfunction or another medical problem. Laboratory tests and physical exams can confirm that you do not suffer from a more complicated medical condition that requires the attention of a physician.

Appreciating Your Mitochondria

Carnitine works its magic on the mitochondria. Virtually every cell in the body has its own energy-producing mitochondria designed to meet the needs of that individual cell. (Mitochondria are not found in the red blood cells or the lens of the eye.) Most cells contain between 500 and 2,000 mitochondria; the highest concentrations of mitochondria exist in the busiest cells of the body, including the brain, heart, kidneys, and other hardworking organs.

While the process of energy production at the cellular level is quite complicated, at the most basic level, it begins when the food we eat is broken down into nutrients (glucose, amino acids, and fatty acids) that can be used as fuel to produce energy. Within the cells, the mitochondria go through a multistep process known as the Krebs cycle to produce adenosine triphosphate (ATP), a chemical that is quite literally the energy source of the body. This ATP is then burned to keep the cells performing their assigned tasks.

To make energy, the mitochondria need to have plenty of carnitine and CoQ10. Carnitine provides the mitochondria with fuel by supplying them with long-chain fatty acids, while CoQ10 helps in the chemical reactions required for energy production. If the cells lack an adequate supply of either carnitine or CoQ10, the mitochondria simply cannot produce enough energy to meet the body's demands. When the body is well stocked with carnitine and CoQ10, the body works efficiently; it spends one ATP molecule to produce three ATP molecules. When stockpiles of carnitine or CoQ10 run low, the mitochondria are less efficient, and they might produce only two ATP molecules for every ATP molecule used, or the body may produce adenosine diphosphate (ADP), which is a less potent fuel. Over time, running your body on cheap fuel will take its toll, damaging the mitochondria and contributing to a growing sense of fatigue.

When our bodies are young, so are our mitochondria. They work tirelessly to produce the abundant energy associated with youth. Over the years, however, our mitochondria age and show signs of wear and tear, just as the rest of

the body does. The mitochondria can grow hard
and less efficient at producing ATP. When the
mitochondria break down, less energy is produced and chronic fatigue sets in. This situation
results in external signs of fatigue such as less
energy to meet the challenge of daily life as well
as internal signs of fatigue—a growing weakness
and inefficiency in the heart, brain, and other organs. This systemic energy crisis can compromise the immune system as a whole, leaving our
bodies more vulnerable to attack from bacteria,
viruses, and other pathogens.

A number of studies have found that people
who suffer from ailments associated with aging—
conditions as varied as cardiovascular disease,
Parkinson's disease, and Alzheimer's disease—
all tend to have abnormally low levels of carnitine and high levels of mitochondria failure.

Don't accept fatigue as a natural consequence
of aging; it is a sign that your body is not producing as much energy as it should. If you pre-
serve and nourish your energy system, your
body will retain a higher level of energy and a
greater state of overall health.

Damage to the Mitochondria

The production of energy in the cells generates
pollution, just as the production of energy at a
coal-fired power plant produces soot and smog.

Within the cells, the production of ATP also results in the production of unwanted, unstable oxygen cells known as free radicals. These free radicals will steal electrons from neighboring cells; they can damage the DNA within a cell and leave the cell susceptible to cancer, heart disease, and many of the symptoms of aging. Unlike other cells, the mitochondria have their own DNA, and free radicals can damage both cellular DNA and mitochondrial DNA.

The body uses antioxidants to neutralize free radicals. The body manufactures its own antioxidants, and we also consume them through the foods we eat and the nutritional supplements we take. As our bodies age, we tend to produce fewer antioxidants, leaving our mitochondria more vulnerable to attack from free radicals—unless, of course, we take steps to fortify the mitochondria by taking carnitine and CoQ10. Both of these substances act as powerful antioxidants, or free radical scavengers.

In addition to acting as an antioxidant, carnitine also helps to protect the mitochondria by preserving their cell membranes. If the mitochondria's membrane, or outer "skin," becomes damaged, it can become difficult for the toxins produced by energy production to escape the mitochondria. These toxins then build up, causing a decline in energy production and the accumulation of still more waste. If enough mitochondria become damaged over time, the cell will no longer perform its assigned function. If enough cells in an organ are damaged, the organ itself will begin to fail, as is common with congestive heart failure.

Mitochondria and Aging

A generation ago, scientists speculated that damage to the mitochondria may be the most important cause of aging and ultimately death. This theory is supported by research that shows that the mitochondria are damaged through so-called deletions as we age; deletions are changes to the genetic code in DNA. Studies on plants, animals, and humans have all shown a link between DNA deletions and signs of aging. Research done at Columbia University found an astounding 10,000-fold increase in DNA deletions in muscle cells of older people, compared to younger folks. Not surprisingly, loss of muscle strength is a common experience associated with aging.

Some organs are more affected by mitochondrial aging than others. The heart and brain appear to be particularly vulnerable to damage, which helps explain why these organs also tend to be particularly responsive to carnitine supplementation. (For information on carnitine and the heart, see Chapter 6; for information on carnitine and the brain, see Chapter 7.)

Some animal studies have demonstrated that

carnitine supplementation can help to reverse the age-related decline in energy. One study done at the University of California, Berkeley, and reported in the 1998 *Proceedings of the National Academy of Sciences* found that supplementation with acetyl-L-carnitine helps restore mitochondrial function in old rats. The researchers spiked the drinking water with acetyl-L-carnitine and gave it to groups of 3- to 5-month-old (young) and 22- to 28-month-old (old) rats for one month. When their liver cells were examined at the end of the supplementation period, the researchers found that the old rats taking the acetyl-L-carnitine experienced a marked improvement in the quality of their mitochondrial membranes. In other words, their mitochondria appeared far more youthful and less damaged than before taking carnitine. (The liver was chosen because the liver stores glycogen, the fuel for the muscles, and it produces bile, which is essential for the metabolism of fat.) This finding is significant because the liver tends to be hard hit by mitochondrial aging; fully two-thirds of the cells in the older livers had dysfunctional mitochondria.

It is also worth noting that the older rats taking acetyl-L-carnitine looked and acted younger. Where their fur was thin and dull before supplementation, it was shiny and fuller after consuming the carnitine. And the once-lethargic and tired rats became much more active physically.

In fact, a computer that recorded their physical activity found that the old rats were just as active physically as rats half their age.

In a third measure of vitality, the rats taking carnitine were found to improve in mental function. Rats, like humans, tend to lose their mental edge as they grow older. The older rats taking acetyl-L-carnitine improved their ability to work through mazes, the quintessential rat intelligence test. What this collection of rat studies demonstrated was truly remarkable: It established a link between the improvement of mitochondrial health in the cells and the improvement in intelligence, appearance, and physical activity in the body.

Carnitine and Chronic Fatigue Syndrome

Carnitine has been shown to be effective in the treatment of chronic fatigue syndrome. Chronic fatigue involves a more severe state of exhaustion than simply feeling tired or rundown; it involves an overwhelming feeling of exhaustion that does not go away with up to a week of rest. While the precise mechanism of the illness is not fully understood, it appears to involve a breakdown in the body's ability to produce energy.

The symptoms of chronic fatigue include reduced mental alertness, depression, lack of motivation, irritability, hostility, indifference, unsociability, uncooperative behavior, lack of personal hygiene, and lack of appetite. Physical symptoms also include recurrent sore throats and infections, sleep disturbances, low-grade fever, headaches, muscle pain and weakness, flu-like symptoms, and lymph node swelling. Using the criteria established by the Centers for Disease Control and Prevention in Atlanta, experts estimate that more than half a million Americans suffer from chronic fatigue syndrome; about 80 percent of those afflicted are women. The symptoms can persist for months or years without abating.

Studies have found that people suffering from chronic fatigue syndrome have low levels of carnitine compared to healthy people. Furthermore, they found that the severity of symptoms tracked the level of carnitine; the lower the levels of carnitine, the more severe the symptoms. By the same token, as people with chronic fatigue syndrome improve, their carnitine levels increase.

In one study, 30 people with chronic fatigue syndrome were given 3 grams of carnitine daily for eight weeks. The longer the people took the carnitine, the more energy they had, and this improvement occurred without negative side effects. The most significant improvement occurred between the fourth and eighth week of the study; if you take carnitine supplements to increase your energy, be sure to take them for at least two months.

For More Information

American Autoimmune Related Diseases Association
Michigan National Bank Building
15475 Gratior
Detroit, MI 48205
(313) 371-8600
www.aarda.org

Chronic Fatigue and Immune Dysfunction Syndrome Association of America
(800) 442-3437
www.cfids.org

Immune Deficiency Foundation
25 West Chesapeake Avenue
Towson, MD 21204
(410) 321-6647
www.primaryimmune.org

FOUR

Achieve Your Personal Best: Carnitine and Sports Performance

WHETHER YOU'RE A WEEKEND ATHLETE, A WELL-trained amateur, or an elite professional, when it comes to the sport of your choice, you want to do your best. As part of your fitness strategy, you may want to join the tens of thousands of athletes of all ability levels who take carnitine supplements to enhance their athletic performance and endurance.

Carnitine helps the body burn fat, and it also helps clear the mitochondria of the waste products created by the generation of energy during exercise. Both functions are necessary for optimal athletic performance. These metabolic benefits can give any athlete an edge, but they offer the greatest advantage to athletes who compete in endurance events. In addition, older athletes often notice the performance-enhancing benefits of carnitine, probably because they tend to have lower levels of carnitine than younger athletes. Also, many studies have found that even elite athletes can benefit from appropriate supplementation.

Carnitine and Endurance

Stored fat is the most abundant source of energy in the body. During a marathon or a long bike ride, an athlete could exercise to the point of depleting the carbohydrate reserves in the muscles, but it would be virtually impossible to exercise long enough to use all of the energy stored in the body's fat reserves. It stands to reason that athletes who are able to utilize energy stored in their fat can exercise longer and harder than those who depend on carbohydrates alone. Since carnitine helps the body burn fat for energy, it can give athletes an edge during athletic training and competition.

A number of studies have shown that carnitine does in fact help athletes work out longer and harder during endurance events. The effects tend to be most dramatic in untrained or out-of-shape athletes, but even well-trained athletes can benefit.

Carnitine and Muscle Damage

Carnitine appears to prevent the muscle damage that can occur during intense exercise and minimize the muscle soreness that can follow a challenging workout. One study of six novice athletes found that those taking 3 grams of carnitine daily for three to six weeks experienced significantly less muscle pain than similar athletes who did not take the supplement.

Carnitine may reduce postexercise tenderness and improve endurance by encouraging the body to use the lactate produced during exercise. Lactate is a by-product of the metabolic process that occurs during exercise; when it accumulates in the muscles, it causes the burning feeling that can cause an athlete to slow down. Because carnitine helps the body burn lactate for fuel, it allows an athlete to work out longer and more strenuously before experiencing symptoms of lactate buildup.

Using Carnitine

Many experts believe that people do not take enough carnitine to experience its full potential for improving sports performance. Some people take 250 milligrams once a day and expect to see performance changes that can be measured with a stopwatch. For most athletes, a dose of 1 to 3 grams is necessary to enhance performance. This dosage is higher than that recommended for most physical conditions because athletic training itself decreases carnitine levels; the higher dose is required to make up for the carnitine excreted in the urine during endurance exercise.

Some experts recommend that athletes divide their dosage between L-carnitine and acetyl-L-carnitine. The L-carnitine form appears to help with the metabolism of fats, while the acetyl-L-carnitine form helps with the metabolism of carbohydrates. By taking both forms, you can take advantage of all that carnitine can do to boost performance.

Athletes should take carnitine on a daily basis for at least four weeks before competition. While the amount of carnitine in the blood peaks about 45 minutes after taking the supplement, the blood level is far less important than the carnitine level in the muscles and cells. It can take several weeks for muscles to be thoroughly saturated with carnitine.

Nutrition for Peak Performance

In addition to carnitine, other nutritional supplements also can help you achieve and maintain the highest level of fitness. As an athlete, good nutrition is essential to your optimal health and performance.

Know Your Nutrients

Scientists have identified approximately 40 different nutrients—including vitamins, essential minerals (needed in relatively large amounts), trace minerals (needed in relatively small amounts), and electrolytes—that are necessary for human health.

Vitamins *are organic substances that the body needs to regulate metabolism, assist in biochemical processes, and prevent disease. Most vitamins are catalysts (or cofactors) in chemical reactions in the body. For example, vitamin B_5 (pantothenic acid) is a cofactor in a series of chemical reactions that burn carbohydrates. Vitamins are either fat soluble or water soluble. As the name implies, fat-soluble vitamins dissolve in the fat; they can be stored by the body for long periods of time and build up to toxic levels if taken in excess. Water-soluble vitamins cannot be stored and must be consumed every day or two; excess levels are eliminated in the urine.*

Minerals *are basic elements; they cannot be manufactured or broken down by living system. However, minerals do combine with vitamins, enzymes, and other substances as part of the essential metabolic processes in the body. While the vitamin content of foods is stable, the mineral content is not. The mineral content of a plant varies from region*

*to region and plant to plant due to variations in the
soil's mineral content.*

Electrolytes *are minerals that allow the transmission of electrical impulses in the body. They also
help to balance the flow of water across the cell
membranes, and they are essential to the maintenance of the balance of the water in the body.*

Athletes have special nutritional require-
ments. The average athlete in training consumes
two or three times more calories than a nonath-
lete. Ideally, an athlete will eat a healthy, balanced diet, but many athletes (and nonathletes)
fall short of their nutritional goals. Even among
people who try to eat a balanced diet, supplements are often necessary to reach optimal levels
of certain nutrients.

A number of books focus on using nutrition
for peak sports performance. The following section provides a brief overview of the essentials
of sports nutrition.

For each nutrient, the listing includes the Performance Daily Intake, an unofficial guideline
developed by sports nutrition researchers to take
into account the higher nutritional needs of athletes. This figure is higher than the Reference
Daily Intakes (RDIs), or recommended nutrient
intakes for healthy adults. The U.S. Food and
Drug Administration has assigned RDIs to 27 vitamins and minerals.

Vitamins

VITAMIN A
Performance Daily Intake: 5,000 to 25,000 IU
(International Units)

Vitamin A helps to form and maintain the healthy function of the eyes, hair, teeth, gums, and mucous membranes; it is also involved in fat metabolism. Vitamin A in animal tissues is called retinol; vitamin A in plants is called beta-carotene. (Beta-carotene is sometimes called a provitamin because it must be broken down by the body into vitamin A before it acts as a vitamin.) Both vitamin A and beta-carotene are antioxidants, which may help protect against cancer and improve resistance to certain diseases.

Strenuous exercise increases the production of free radicals, molecules that are missing an electron. These cells pull electrons from other molecules, causing cellular damage. The body attempts to offset the problem by producing antioxidant enzymes. Supplemental antioxidants, such as vitamin A, can help prevent muscle and tissue damage, especially during endurance exercise.

SIGNS OF DEFICIENCY: Night blindness, retarded growth in children, impaired resistance to disease, infection, rough skin, dry eyes.

SIGNS OF OVERDOSE: Headaches, blurred vision, skin rash, extreme fatigue, diarrhea, nausea, loss of appetite, hair loss, menstrual irregularities, liver damage, dizziness.

GOOD FOOD SOURCES: Whole milk, butter, fortified margarine, eggs, green leafy and yellow vegetables and fruits, organ meats, cheese, and fish.

VITAMIN B$_1$ (THIAMINE)
Performance Daily Intake: 30 to 300 milligrams

Vitamin B$_1$ is necessary for carbohydrate metabolism; it promotes normal appetite and digestion; it is needed for nerve function.

Studies have found that taking increased doses of thiamine three to five days before an endurance athletic event may improve performance. Another study has found that vitamin B$_1$ may help improve the accuracy of firing among sharpshooters and marksmen.

SIGNS OF DEFICIENCY: Anxiety, hysteria, nausea, memory loss, irritability, depression, muscle cramps, loss of appetite; in extreme cases, beriberi, paralysis, and heart failure.

SIGNS OF OVERDOSE: Unknown; however, due to the interdependency of the B-complex vitamins, an excess of one may cause a deficiency of another.

GOOD FOOD SOURCES: Pork, poultry, liver, pasta, wheat germ, whole-grain or enriched breads, lima beans, seafood, nuts, seeds.

WARNING: Antibiotics, sulfa drugs, and oral contraceptives may decrease thiamine levels in the body; eating a high-carbohydrate diet may increase the need for thiamine.

VITAMIN B_2 (RIBOFLAVIN)
Performance Daily Intake: 30 to 300 milligrams

Vitamin B_2 assists in the metabolism of carbohydrates, proteins, and fats; it helps maintain good vision.

Vitamin B_2 has been reported to improve overall athletic performance by improving muscle excitability.

SIGNS OF DEFICIENCY: Lesions around the nose and eyes; sores on the lips, mouth, and tongue; intolerance of light.

SIGNS OF OVERDOSE: Same as for vitamin B_1.

GOOD FOOD SOURCES: Milk, cheese, fish, eggs, green leafy vegetables, liver, meat, whole-grain or.enriched breads and cereals, bee pollen, nuts, wheat germ.

WARNING: Using oral contraceptives and exercising strenuously increase the need for riboflavin.

VITAMIN B_3 (NIACIN)
Performance Daily Intake: 20 to 100 milligrams

Vitamin B_3 promotes normal appetite and digestion; it is needed for general metabolic activity.

The role of vitamin B_3 on exercise depends on your sport. Studies indicate that vitamin B_3 may improve performance of power athletes who need quick bursts of energy because these athletes obtain their energy from glycogen, and vitamin B_3 appears to speed the release of glycogen from the muscles. On the other hand, vitamin B_3 seems to impair the performance of endurance athletes because the speedy depletion of glycogen causes early fatigue. Research on the use of vitamin B_3 among athletes is ongoing.

SIGNS OF DEFICIENCY: Irritability, memory loss, headaches, skin disorders.

SIGNS OF OVERDOSE: Ulcers, liver disorders, high blood sugar levels, high uric acid levels, depression.

GOOD FOOD SOURCES: Liver, meat, fish, poultry, green vegetables, nuts, whole-grain or enriched breads and cereals (except corn).

WARNING: Niacin should not be used in large amounts by people suffering from gout, peptic ulcers, glaucoma, liver disease, or diabetes.

VITAMIN B_5
Performance Daily Intake: 25 to 200 milligrams

Vitamin B_5 is needed for the metabolism of carbohydrates, fats, and proteins; it is also needed for the formation of certain hormones.

Vitamin B_5 supports the release of energy from carbohydrates and fatty acids. Some studies have supported the use of vitamin B_5 by endurance athletes the week prior to competition to improve performance.

SIGNS OF DEFICIENCY: Fatigue, numbness, emotional swings.

SIGNS OF OVERDOSE: May increase the need for thiamine (vitamin B_1) and lead to thiamine deficiency.

GOOD FOOD SOURCES: Found in most animal and plant foods, also produced by intestinal bacteria.

VITAMIN B$_6$
Performance Daily Intake: 20 to 100 milligrams

Vitamin B$_6$ assists in the metabolism of proteins, carbohydrates, and fats; it also aids in the formation of red blood cells and the functioning of the nervous system and brain. Studies have found that vitamin B$_6$'s impact on athletic performance strongly resembles that of vitamin B$_3$.

SIGNS OF DEFICIENCY: Depression, confusion, convulsions, irritability, insomnia, reduced resistance to infection, sores in the mouth, itchy skin.

SIGNS OF OVERDOSE: Overdose can lead to dependency and cause signs of deficiency when intake is reduced to normal levels.

GOOD FOOD SOURCES: Green leafy vegetables, meat, fish, poultry, whole-grain cereals, liver, nuts, seeds, bananas, avocados, and potatoes.

WARNING: Antidepressants, estrogen, and oral contraceptives may increase the need for vitamin B$_6$.

VITAMIN B$_{12}$
Performance Daily Intake: 12 to 200 micrograms

Vitamin B$_{12}$ is necessary for the formation of genetic material and red blood cells. It is considered a major "energy vitamin"; it is commonly used by athletes to enhance their performance. It has been shown to improve growth in children with growth disorders. Athletes report that it raises energy levels and increases appetite.

SIGNS OF DEFICIENCY: Pernicious anemia.

SIGNS OF OVERDOSE: Same as for vitamin B$_1$.

GOOD FOOD SOURCES: Milk, saltwater fish, oysters, meat, liver, kidneys, eggs, pork, cheese, and yogurt.

WARNING: Antigout medications, anticoagulant drugs and potassium supplements may block the absorption of vitamin B$_{12}$.

BIOTIN (VITAMIN H)
Performance Daily Intake: 125 to 300 micrograms

Biotin is involved in the formation of certain fatty acids and in the metabolism of carbohydrates and fats. It promotes the development of healthy hair, skin, sweat glands, nerve tissue, and bone marrow.

SIGNS OF DEFICIENCY: Depression, insomnia, muscle pain, anemia (rare except in infants).

SIGNS OF OVERDOSE: Same as for vitamin B_1.

GOOD FOOD SOURCES: Eggs, green leafy vegetables, liver, string beans, milk, meat, nuts.

WARNING: Consuming saccharin can inhibit biotin absorption.

FOLATE (FOLIC ACID)
Performance Daily Intake: 400 to 1,200 micrograms

Folate assists in the formation of certain proteins and genetic materials as well as in the formation of red blood cells. In general, athletes benefit from higher-than-average folate intake; weight lifters and bodybuilders tend to recover faster from their workouts and experience faster growth rates when taking supplemental folate.

SIGNS OF DEFICIENCY: Impaired cell division, creation of abnormal red blood cells, anemia, and mental problems.

SIGNS OF OVERDOSE: Gastrointestinal distress, insomnia, malaise.

GOOD FOOD SOURCES: Green leafy vegetables, liver, kidney, avocados, wheat germ, legumes, brain, and nuts.

WARNING: Use of oral contraceptives may increase the need for folic acid; inadequate intake early in pregnancy increases the risk of spina bifida in the infant.

VITAMIN C
Performance Daily Intake: 800 to 3,000 milligrams

Vitamin C helps bind cells together and strengthen the walls of the blood vessels; it helps fight infections and promotes wound healing. A number of studies have found that, for athletes, vitamin C can help increase strength, reduce lactic acid buildup, and allow the body to use glycogen more efficiently.

SIGNS OF DEFICIENCY: Scurvy, bleeding gums, loose teeth, slow healing, dry and rough skin, loss of appetite.

SIGNS OF OVERDOSE: Bladder and kidney stones, urinary tract irritations, diarrhea; overconsumption can led to dependency, which can cause deficiency symptoms when intake is reduced to normal levels.

GOOD FOOD SOURCES: Citrus fruits and juices, green leafy vegetables, tomatoes, red and green peppers, melons, cauliflower, strawberries, and new potatoes.

WARNING: Aspirin, alcohol, analgesics, antidepressants, anticoagulants, oral contraceptives, and steroids may reduce vitamin C levels in the body.

VITAMIN D
Performance Daily Intake: 400 to 1,000 IU

Vitamin D is needed for the body to absorb and metabolize calcium and phosphorus to build bones and teeth. There is some evidence to support claims that vitamin D helps improve muscle strength, prevent low calcium levels, and enhance immunity.

SIGNS OF DEFICIENCY: Rickets in children, thin bones in adults.

SIGNS OF OVERDOSE: Calcium deposits in the body, nausea, loss of appetite, kidney stones, high blood pressure, high cholesterol levels, and fragile bones.

GOOD FOOD SOURCES: Fortified milk, liver, fish liver and fish oils, egg yolks, butter; exposure to the sun's ultraviolet rays enables the body to produce its own vitamin D.

WARNING: Vitamin D should not be taken without calcium; intestinal disorders, liver problems, and gallbladder disease can interfere with the absorption of vitamin D.

VITAMIN E
Performance Daily Intake: 200 to 1,000 IU

Vitamin E helps the body form red blood cells, muscles, and other tissues; it is necessary for the breakdown of fats. Studies have found that taking 200 to 1,200 IU of vitamin E can help athletes by improving energy production, reducing cellular damage, maintaining muscle tissue, and helping testosterone production.

SIGNS OF DEFICIENCY: Deficiency is rare except in people with an impaired absorption of fat.

SIGNS OF OVERDOSE: Not clearly understood.

GOOD FOOD SOURCES: Wheat germ, vegetable oils, margarine, nuts, seeds, eggs, milk, whole-grain cereals, and breads.

WARNING: People with diabetes, thyroid disease, or heart disease should not take high doses of vitamin E.

VITAMIN K
Performance Daily Intake: 80 to 180 micrograms

Vitamin K is needed for normal blood clotting and bone metabolism. Athletes often take supplemental vitamin K to reverse the tissue damage they experience during training.

SIGNS OF DEFICIENCY: Bleeding disorders and liver damage.

SIGNS OF OVERDOSE: Jaundice in infants; unknown in adults.

GOOD FOOD SOURCES: Green leafy vegetables, peas, cereals, dairy products, liver, potatoes, cabbage, wheat germ, tomatoes, eggs; it is also produced by intestinal bacteria.

WARNING: Antibiotics can interfere with the absorption of vitamin K.

Minerals

BORON
Performance Daily Intake: 6 to 12 milligrams

Boron is a trace mineral that plays a role in the metabolism of calcium, phosphorus, and magnesium; it also affects parathyroid-hormone action and bone formation. Athletes use boron because it is believed to increase testosterone production. According to a 1987 study, supplemental boron increased testosterone levels in postmenopausal women. Another study done in 1992 found that bodybuilders who took 2.5 milligrams of boron daily did not show signs of increased testosterone levels or strength.

SIGNS OF DEFICIENCY: Boron deficiency has never been reported in humans; it is needed in such small quantities that it is easily obtained in the diet.

SIGNS OF OVERDOSE: Nausea, vomiting, diarrhea, dermatitis, nervous system irritability, kidney failure.

GOOD FOOD SOURCES: Green leafy vegetables, fruits, nuts, and grains.

CALCIUM
Performance Daily Intake: 1,200 to 2,600 milligrams

Calcium helps build strong bones and teeth; it helps blood clot and helps nerve and muscle function. Recent research indicates that calcium supplements can reduce the risk of high blood pressure in pregnant women. Fully 99 percent of the body's calcium is stored in the skeleton. Taking supplemental calcium along with regular exercise can strengthen bone density.

SIGNS OF DEFICIENCY: Rickets in children, osteoporosis in adults.

SIGNS OF OVERDOSE: Drowsiness, calcium deposits, impaired absorption of iron and other minerals.

GOOD FOOD SOURCES: Milk and milk products, cheese, green leafy vegetables, citrus fruits, dried peas and beans, sardines (with bones), shellfish, whole-grain breads.

WARNING: People with kidney stones or kidney disease should not take calcium supplements; too much calcium can interfere with the absorption of zinc.

CHROMIUM
Performance Daily Intake: 200 to 600 micrograms

Chromium is a trace mineral that is necessary for blood-sugar regulation. Chromium is an important cofactor for energy production as well as for tissue growth and repair. Several studies have shown that taking supplemental chromium can help increase the rate of muscle gain and fat loss among athletes in training.

SIGNS OF DEFICIENCY: Infertility, cloudy corneas, atherosclerosis.

SIGNS OF OVERDOSE: Chronic exposure to chromium dust in industry has been linked to lung cancer.

GOOD FOOD SOURCES: Brewer's yeast, oysters, eggs, whole grains.

COPPER
Performance Daily Intake: 3 to 6 milligrams

Copper is a trace mineral necessary for the maintenance of healthy blood cells and bones. Copper also plays an important role in energy production; it is a necessary part of the enzyme cytochrome oxidase, which is essential for energy production.

SIGNS OF DEFICIENCY: Anemia, elevated cholesterol levels, infertility.

SIGNS OF OVERDOSE: Nausea, vomiting, muscle aches, stomach pains.

GOOD FOOD SOURCES: Liver, kidneys, nuts, shellfish, legumes, yeast, cocoa, whole-grain cereals.

WARNING: High levels of zinc and vitamin C can reduce copper levels.

IODINE
Performance Daily Intake: 200 to 400 micrograms

Iodine is necessary for the normal function of the thyroid gland. The thyroid helps regulate metabolism, energy production, growth, and overall physical performance.

SIGNS OF DEFICIENCY: Thyroid enlargement.

SIGNS OF OVERDOSE: Poisoning.

GOOD FOOD SOURCES: Iodized salt, seafood, fish liver oil.

WARNING: People with hypothyroid disorder should avoid high-iodine foods; when eaten in large amounts, some raw foods (Brussels sprouts, cabbage, kale, peaches, spinach) can block the uptake of iodine into the thyroid.

IRON
Performance Daily Intake: 25 to 60 milligrams

Iron combines with protein to make hemoglobin (which carries oxygen in the blood) and myoglobin (which stores oxygen in the muscles). Female athletes, endurance athletes, and athletes on low-calorie diets are especially prone to iron deficiency.

SIGNS OF DEFICIENCY: Anemia, weakness, fatigue, headache, shortness of breath.

SIGNS OF OVERDOSE: Buildup in the liver, pancreas, and heart.

GOOD FOOD SOURCES: Liver, red meat, egg yolks, shellfish, green leafy vegetables, peas, beans, dried prunes, raisins, apricots, whole-grain and enriched breads and cereals, and nuts.

WARNING: High amounts of zinc and vitamin E can interfere with iron absorption; tannins (found in tea) can also inhibit iron absorption.

MAGNESIUM
Performance Daily Intake: 400 to 800 milligrams

Magnesium is necessary for the metabolism of protein and carbohydrates. Researchers have found that athletes in training, especially endurance athletes, often deplete their magnesium stores.

SIGNS OF DEFICIENCY: Muscle tremors, leg cramps, weakness, irregular heartbeat, constipation.

SIGNS OF OVERDOSE: Upset in the calcium-magnesium ratio, resulting in impaired nervous system function; especially dangerous in people with impaired kidney function.

GOOD FOOD SOURCES: Raw leafy green vegetables, nuts, soybeans, whole-grain breads and cereals, and shrimp.

WARNING: Consumption of alcohol, diuretics, and high amounts of zinc and vitamin D all increase the body's needs for magnesium.

MANGANESE
Performance Daily Intake: 15 to 45 milligrams

Manganese is necessary for tendon and bone formation, nervous system function, and fat and vitamin metabolism. It is also a critical part of enzymes that aid in the formation of bone and connective tissue. Manganese can be helpful to athletes in the prevention of injury and in recovery following strenuous exercise; it is also an antioxidant, so it can help to prevent cellular damage caused by exercise.

SIGNS OF DEFICIENCY: Cartilage problems, infertility, birth defects.

SIGNS OF OVERDOSE: Irritability, muscle tremors.

GOOD FOOD SOURCES: Bran, coffee, tea, nuts, beans, and peas.

MOLYBDENUM
Performance Daily Intake: 100 to 300 micrograms

Molybdenum is a trace mineral that is present in a number of enzymes involved in energy production, nitrogen metabolism, and uric-acid formation.

SIGNS OF DEFICIENCY: Molybdenum deficiency has never been reported in a human because the mineral is required in such small amounts.

SIGNS OF OVERDOSE: Gout, growth disorders, lowered copper levels.

GOOD FOOD SOURCES: Milk, beans, bread, cereal, and organ meats.

PHOSPHORUS
Performance Daily Intake: 800 to 1,600 milligrams

Phosphorus helps build bones and teeth; it is needed to change food into energy. Scientists have long appreciated the importance of phosphorus in energy production. During World War I, German troops were given phosphorus supplements to reduce fatigue and improve their physical performance. Recent studies have confirmed the benefits of using phosphorus supplements, especially among endurance athletes.

SIGNS OF DEFICIENCY: Weakness, bone pain, decreased appetite, anemia.

SIGNS OF OVERDOSE: Upset in calcium-phosphorus ratio, hindering uptake of calcium, which can show up as osteoporosis or weak, brittle bones.

GOOD FOOD SOURCES: Meat, poultry, fish, eggs, dried peas and beans, milk and milk products, egg yolk, phosphates in processed foods and soft drinks.

WARNING: Excess phosphorus can interfere with calcium uptake.

POTASSIUM
Performance Daily Intake: 2,500 to 4,000
milligrams

Potassium plays a critical role in the fluid balance; it also functions in nerve transmission, muscle contraction, and glycogen formation. If you do not eat many fruits and vegetables, be sure to take supplemental potassium. In addition, if you train for long hours (especially in hot climates) or if you sweat excessively, you should be sure to take extra potassium.

SIGNS OF DEFICIENCY: Muscle weakness, irritability, irregular heartbeat, kidney and lung failure.

SIGNS OF OVERDOSE: cardiac irregularities.

GOOD FOOD SOURCES: Bananas, dried fruits, peanut butter, potatoes, orange juice, fruits and vegetables, milk, and beef.

SELENIUM
Performance Daily Intake: 100 to 300 micrograms

Selenium works with vitamin E in the break-down of fat in the body; it is necessary for healthy liver, heart, and white blood cells. Selenium is a powerful antioxidant; it can help shorten recovery time and minimize tissue damage during exercise.

SIGNS OF DEFICIENCY: Liver disease, skin problems, arthritis.

SIGNS OF OVERDOSE: Unknown.

GOOD FOOD SOURCES: Seafood, egg yolks, chicken, meat, garlic, whole-grain cereals, brewer's yeast, fish, and organ meats.

SODIUM
Performance Daily Intake: 1,500 to 4,500 milligrams

Sodium helps maintain water balance inside and outside the cells; it is involved in nerve and muscle function. Athletes have higher sodium demands due to their excessive sweating during exercise; supplementation may be required, depending on the sodium content of the diet.

SIGNS OF DEFICIENCY: Water retention, muscle cramps, headache, weakness, exhaustion, and nausea.

SIGNS OF OVERDOSE: High blood pressure, kidney disease, congestive heart failure.

GOOD FOOD SOURCES: Salt, processed foods, ham, meat, fish, poultry, eggs, milk, and salted crackers.

WARNING: High sodium levels may result in potassium deficiency and liver and kidney disease.

ZINC
Performance Daily Intake: 15 to 60 milligrams

Zinc is necessary for the red blood cells to move carbon dioxide away from the tissues; it is involved in the metabolism of carbohydrates and vitamins. Low zinc intake is common, especially among endurance athletes, power athletes, female athletes, and athletes on low-calorie diets. Supplemental zinc can improve performance by increasing muscle endurance.

SIGNS OF DEFICIENCY: Loss of taste, delayed wound healing, infertility.

SIGNS OF OVERDOSE: Nausea, vomiting, abdominal pain.

GOOD FOOD SOURCES: Meats, fish, egg yolk, milk, oysters, whole grains, nuts, and legumes.

WARNING: Drinking "hard" (mineral-laden) water can upset zinc levels.

Metabolites

Metabolites are substances that take part in metabolism. They can come from food sources or supplements, or they can be produced by the body as part of the metabolic process.

BIOFLAVONOIDS
Performance Daily Intake: 200 to 2,000 milligrams

The bioflavonoids are naturally occurring plant compounds that improve the absorption of vitamin C. They also strengthen the capillary walls and have an anti-inflammatory effect.

SIGNS OF DEFICIENCY: Bioflavonoid deficiency has not been established in humans.

SIGNS OF OVERDOSE: Unknown.

GOOD FOOD SOURCES: Citrus fruits, grapes, plums, apricots, cherries, blackberries, and rose hips.

CHOLINE
Performance Daily Intake: 600 to 1,200 milligrams

Choline is often considered part of the B-complex family. It is involved in fatty-acid metabolism and in the prevention of fat deposits in the liver. It is also used by the body to make neurotransmitters for brain function.

SIGNS OF DEFICIENCY: Choline deficiency is not usually seen in humans since choline is present in the diet.

SIGNS OF OVERDOSE: Diarrhea, depression, and dizziness.

GOOD FOOD SOURCES: Egg yolks, liver, soybeans, fatty food, meat, whole grains, asparagus, green beans, spinach, and wheat germ.

INOSITOL
Performance Daily Intake: 800 to 1,200 milligrams

Inositol is sometimes classified as a member of the B-complex family. It is more accurately called myo-inositol. Inositol assists in the metabolism of fatty acids and carbohydrates; it also assists in calcium absorption.

SIGNS OF DEFICIENCY: Buildup of fat in the liver that may affect the nervous system.

SIGNS OF OVERDOSE: None known.

GOOD FOOD SOURCES: Whole grains, fruits, milk, nuts, meat, and vegetables.

Smart Shopping for Supplements

The regular use of carnitine, CoQ10, and other supplements can be expensive. When shopping for supplements, consider the following tips.

- *Look for store brands.* All vitamins are essentially the same, so forget the brand names and look for the bargain. If you buy a heavily advertised product, all you're doing is paying for the advertising.
- *For the most part, don't worry about going "natural."* The body uses both natural and synthetic vitamins in the same way. The big difference is cost: It would take tons of food to extract all the vitamins used in nutrition supplements. Supplements produced in the laboratory are chemically identical—and much cheaper to produce. One exception: vitamin E. Natural vita-

min E is absorbed better than the synthetic version.

- *Check the expiration date.* Nutrition supplements lose potency over time. Also, to be sure to store them in a cool, dry place.
- *Don't pay more for "chelated" minerals.* Some manufacturers sell supplements that they claim can be absorbed by the body more easily because the minerals have been chelated, or attached to an amino acid. There is no evidence to support this claim, although chelated minerals do cost more.

FIVE

Burn Up the Fat:
Carnitine and Weight Loss

TWO OUT OF THREE AMERICANS ARE OVERWEIGHT, according to national surveys, and one out of three is obese (or more than 20 percent above ideal weight). Over the years those extra pounds take a toll on overall health, contributing to heart disease, diabetes, high blood pressure, gallstones, and some types of cancer. In fact, experts believe that obesity and weight problems contribute to more than 300,000 deaths a year. Fortunately, lowering your weight can lower your risk of developing these life-threatening conditions—and carnitine can help.

Carnitine helps the body burn fat for energy, depleting the fat reserves throughout the body. Carnitine is essential for weight loss; fat cannot be "burned" for fuel unless carnitine transports it to the mitochondria or energy centers of the cells. If carnitine levels drop, the mitochondria become less efficient at burning fat, and overall energy levels drop. As a result, carnitine deficiency can lead to weight gain and obesity.

To lose weight, you need to be sure your cells have plenty of carnitine available to meet the demands of the mitochondria. Many people tend to put on extra pounds in midlife, which is the same time that carnitine supplies begin to drop off and metabolism slows. Taking supplemental carnitine helps the body burn fat and produce more energy, which can help keep off unwanted pounds. Because energy levels remain higher, many people find it easier to exercise and remain physically active, which in turn helps the body burn additional fat. To maintain your optimal weight, you need to maintain optimal nutrition, including sufficient levels of carnitine.

Are You Overweight?

While all the experts agree that too much body fat is hazardous to your health, there is little consensus on how much fat is too much. Ten years ago the federal government's suggested weight charts allowed for wide variations in weight. These charts also established a separate and more liberal set of standards for people over age 35, sending a clear message that putting on a little weight during middle age would not necessarily hurt you.

Not so, concluded the Nurses Health Study several years later. This 15-year study of 100,000 nurses found that the healthiest weights were 15 percent below the U.S. averages.

Then, in late 1995, the federal government released a new set of guidelines that, as the table shows, falls between those extremes.

Healthy Weight Ranges for Men and Women

DIETARY GUIDELINES FOR AMERICANS, 1995

HEIGHT	WEIGHT (in pounds)
4'10"	91–119
4'11"	94–124
5'0"	97–128
5'1"	101–132
5'2"	104–137
5'3"	107–141
5'4"	111–146
5'5"	114–150
5'6"	118–155

5'7"	121–160
5'8"	125–164
5'9"	129–169
5'10"	132–174
5'11"	136–179
6'0"	140–184
6'1"	144–189
6'2"	148–195
6'3"	152–200
6'4"	156–205
6'5"	160–211
6'6"	164–216

This table provides a good basic guide, as long as you keep in mind that the weights apply to all ages and offer a 30- to 40-pound range of acceptable, healthy weights for any given height. (Still, the upper end of the range on this table is about 10 to 15 pounds lighter than the 1990 version.)

Another way to assess your weight is to calculate your body mass index (BMI). To determine your BMI, multiply your weight (in pounds) by 705. Divide the result by your height (in inches). Now divide that result by your height again. Regardless of age, most healthy adults have a body mass index in the 20s. The risk of premature death rises as your body mass index rises above 25.

Whether you assess your weight using the height-weight tables or the body mass index, remember that the higher your weight or ratio climbs above the healthy range, the higher your risk of developing weight-related illnesses.

Still, pounds alone don't tell the whole story. One critical issue is where those pounds are located. Fat around your middle—in the abdomen and chest—is much more hazardous than fat around your hips, thighs, and buttocks. (As a rule, it's also much easier to lose.) Abdominal fat enters the bloodstream more easily than fat from the lower body, raising cholesterol levels and increasing the risk of cardiovascular disease.

A quick look in the mirror can show you where you tend to pack on the pounds. Researchers have found that a waist measurement of more than 34 inches in women or 40 inches in men strongly correlates with other indications of obesity. If you want a more sophisticated assessment, you can calculate your waist-to-hip ratio. To do this, measure your waist (in inches) at its narrowest point; then measure your hips at their widest point. Divide the waist measurement by the hip measurement. Women should have a ratio of less than 0.8; men, less than 1.0. A higher ratio indicates that you have too much abdominal fat and you should make an effort to lose weight, regardless of where your weight falls on the weight tables.

Beyond the Scales

Of course, weight matters, but do not ignore the importance of regular exercise. While researchers often focus on the link between overweight and longevity, recent research has demonstrated the critical role of exercise. Epidemiologist Steven Blair and his colleagues at the Cooper Institute for Aerobics Research in Dallas followed 25,000 men and found that among those who exercised regularly, the fat ones lived as long as the thin ones. And interestingly, the thin men who were out of shape were three times more likely to die than the overweight men who got regular exercise. In other words, exercise may be even more important than weight in determining who lives longest. Fat or thin, we all need to exercise regularly. Carnitine helps on both fronts: it provides additional energy for exercise and helps the body burn unwanted fat.

Exercise can also help you lose weight. Whatever type you choose, exercise increases your basal metabolic rate (the number of calories your body burns at rest), allowing your body to burn more calories even when you're sitting still. Studies have found that all it takes is 30 minutes of steady exercise to boost the metabolic rate for at least 12 hours.

In addition, the muscle mass you build through exercise further revs your metabolic engine, since muscle burns more calories than fat, even when at rest. (A pound of muscle burns about 45 calories a day, compared to a pound of fat, which burns fewer than 2 calories a day.) While low-calorie diets can lower your metabolism, exercise can stoke your metabolism, making it easier to lose weight.

Eat to Lose

If you need to lose weight, remember that weight loss should be slow and steady. If you try to drop more than a pound or two a week (either through diet or exercise), your body will switch into its fat-preservation mode and fight to keep you as plump as possible. Mother Nature designed us that way: Whenever the human body loses too much weight too fast, hormones cause the metabolism to slow down and hunger pangs to kick in to prevent us from wasting away (no matter how fat we are).

Alas, there are no magic formulas or weight-loss secrets that will make the task of losing weight quick and painless. The truth is that to lose weight—and to keep it off—you must change the harmful habits that made you fat in the first place. You must commit yourself to eating a well-balanced diet and getting regular exercise. Carnitine can help the body burn fat, but it can't make up for a life of excess.

Eating right doesn't mean that you must swear off all your favorite foods and become a martyr to the cause. In fact, drastic measure almost always fail. Instead, keep the following tips in mind:

- **Calories do count**. While it is unnecessary and frustrating to count every calorie, you do need to monitor your calories rather than simply watch the fat intake. To figure out how many calories you can eat per day and lose about one pound a week, multiply your current weight by 10, then add 100 calories. For example, if you weigh 160 pounds, you can average about 1,700 calories each day and still lose one pound a week. Remember, cutting calories too much can undermine your diet by slowing your metabolism and making matters even worse.

- **Say yes to fiber**. A high-fiber diet keeps the digestive system moving; it helps prevent certain types of cancer; and it fills you up, so you'll be less tempted to snack on less healthful fare.
- **Add flavor to your life**. Not with fat but with herbs, spices, and other seasonings. If low-fat foods taste bland and uninspired, punch them up with a trip to the spice rack.
- **Don't forget the most important meal of the day**. They're all important, but breakfast can be especially helpful in switching your body from the sleep mode into the high-energy mode. If you skip breakfast, you'll drag through the morning (metabolically as well as in mood), and you'll be more likely to overeat later in the day.
- **Don't skip other meals either**. Breakfast isn't the only meal you shouldn't skip. Skipping lunch or dinner can also cause your metabolic rate to drop. You will gain more weight if you eat a single 2,100-calorie meal each day than if you eat three 700-calorie meals. By spreading your calorie throughout the day, you can actually eat up to 20 percent more calories without gaining weight.
- **Try to maintain a stable weight.** Your body doesn't like to experience large fluctuations

in weight, so it will strive to return your weight to its perceived "normal" point. After you lose weight, your body produces enzymes that encourage the regaining of fat, and the fat is regained more readily with each major shift in weight. Some researchers suspect that this new fat tends to accumulate around the middle, the pattern associated with the highest risk of weight-related health problems.

For More Information

Nutrition Education Association
P.O. Box 20301
3647 Glen Haven
Houston, TX 77225
(713) 665-2946

Nutrition for Optimal Health
P.O. Box 380
Winnetka, IL 60093
(708) 786-5326

SIX

Heart of the Matter: Carnitine and Heart Health

YOUR HEART AND CIRCULATORY SYSTEM FEED every cell in your body with life-giving oxygen. This complex 12,400-mile network of arteries, veins, and blood vessels circulates blood from your heart to the farthest reaches of your body. In a healthy adult, the heart beats about 100,000 times a day, pumping the equivalent of more than 4,000 gallons of blood. That's an impressive accomplishment—one that underscores the importance of maintaining a well-tuned heart and circulatory system.

But all too often the system fails. Heart disease is the leading cause of death in the United States; it is responsible for one out of every five deaths. Heart attacks, atherosclerosis, (formation of cholesterol plaque in the arteries), congestive heart failure, strokes, and other circulatory diseases claim about 1 million lives a year. In addition, a huge number of Americans—more than 63 million—live with some form of heart or blood vessel disease.

The heart requires an unending supply of energy to keep pumping effectively. Because carnitine is crucial for fat burning and energy production, the heart needs an adequate supply of carnitine to work its best. Low levels of carnitine can compromise heart health. By the same token, optimal levels of carnitine can help prevent many forms of cardiovascular disease.

Carnitine and the Mitochondria

Heart health is directly linked to the health of the mitochondria. The heart depends on the mitochondria to provide it with the energy required to beat steadily and rhythmically 24 hours a day for a lifetime. In turn, the mitochondria depend on carnitine to maintain a supply of long-chain fatty acids to burn. As long as there is a sufficient supply of carnitine to satisfy the demands of the mitochondria, the system works well. When carnitine supplies diminish in mid-life, the energy system slows and problems begin to arise.

Carnitine deficiency can damage the mitochondria by allowing toxins to accumulate in the cells. As discussed earlier, carnitine helps to remove the toxic by-products of energy production from the mitochondria. When the body lacks a sufficient supply of carnitine to perform this task, the toxins build up in the cells and damage the mitochondria. When the mitochondria are damaged, they no longer work as efficiently, and energy production is reduced. Over time, the collective damage to the mitochondria can reduce heart function, leading to heart disease.

Not surprisingly, studies have found that people suffering from heart disease tend to have more problems with their mitochondria. In addition, because the mitochondria become lethargic and carnitine shuttles fewer fatty acids to the cells for fuel, these fats accumulate in the blood, where they contribute to cardiovascular disease.

Taking carnitine and CoQ10 can help protect the mitochondria as well as the heart. People suffering from heart disease tend to have abnormally low levels of carnitine, although supplementation can restore carnitine to desirable levels.

To find out whether carnitine can help to restore the mitochondria and strengthen the heart, researchers in Italy administered acetyl-L-carnitine to a group of rats. When the rats' hearts were removed and analyzed, the scientists found that their mitochondria were healthy and youthful, compared to a second group of rats that did not receive the acetyl-L-carnitine. Specifically, they found that the carnitine-treated mitochondria had higher levels of an enzyme required for energy production and that the mitochondria had stronger cell membranes. In sum, the carnitine-treated hearts had maintained superior mitochondrial function compared to the group that did not receive the supplement.

Animal studies have found that carnitine deficiency takes its toll on heart health over time. Researchers gave young male rats a drug to create mild carnitine deficiency. After 24 to 36 weeks, the heart function of the carnitine-deprived rats was tested. The rats' hearts performed well under normal conditions, but when stressed, they could not meet the more strenuous energy demands.

If this finding in laboratory rats has some bearing on healthy humans, then, over time, a mild carnitine deficiency could lead to significant cardiovascular problems over the years. By the same token, supplementation with carnitine could help to keep the mitochondria functioning well and help ward off heart disease.

How Carnitine Heals the Heart

A number of studies have found that carnitine can help to control or reverse heart disease in several of its many forms. Consider the following evidence involving carnitine supplementation and certain types of heart disease.

Angina. The pain may start with constriction in the center of the chest, then it radiates to the throat, back, neck, jaw, and down the left arm.

You break into a sweat, struggle for breath, and feel nauseated and dizzy. You may assume you're in the throes of a full-blown heart attack, but within 10 minutes or so, it's over, and the pain gradually subsides. What you've experienced is not a heart attack but an attack of angina pectoris.

Angina is a symptom that the heart has been damaged. Most attacks come after the heart is stressed, either through physical or emotional excitement. Angina is caused by coronary artery disease, particularly atherosclerosis. The best way to manage angina is to keep the heart and circulatory system as healthy as possible.

Carnitine is one of the most important nutritional supplements used to treat angina. In fact, angina patients often respond so well to the use of carnitine that sometimes they can scale back on the amount of heart medication they take. One of the ways researchers measure the effectiveness of an angina treatment is to assess how much physical exercise (stress) a person with angina can endure before experiencing an attack of angina. As part of one clinical trial done in Japan, people given 900 mg of carnitine daily were able to increase their exercise load by fully 10 percent. Another trial involved a higher dose of carnitine—2 grams daily. The angina sufferers were able to increase their exercise tolerance by an average of 22 percent.

Heart attack. The heart is a muscle, and like any other muscle, it needs oxygen to stay alive. When all or part of the heart muscle dies due to lack of oxygen, it is called a heart attack, or myocardial infarction. Each year more than 1.5 million Americans suffer heart attacks, and about one out of three of them dies.

Many heart attacks are caused by blood clots. When blood flows through an artery of the heart that has been narrowed by atherosclerosis, it slows down and tends to clot. When the clot becomes big enough, it cuts off the blood supply to the portion of the heart muscle below the clot, and that part of the heart muscle begins to die.

Heart attack also can occur when the heartbeat becomes irregular. In severe cases, this condition, known as arrhythmia, can prevent sufficient blood from reaching the heart muscle.

Carnitine has been found to prevent future heart attacks and extend the life expectancy of people who suffered heart attacks. In one 1992 study of 160 people who had experienced a previous heart attack, half were given 4 grams of carnitine daily for a year, and the other were given a placebo. The group receiving carnitine experienced improved heart rates and rhythms and had a significantly lower mortality rate compared to the placebo group.

Another study done four years later found similar benefits in patients given just 2 grams of carnitine daily for 28 days. In fact, both the number of subsequent heart attacks and the death rates in the group taking carnitine were half the rate of the people in the control group.

When administered immediately following the episode, carnitine also can minimize the damage of a heart attack. Research published in the *Journal of the American College of Cardiology* in 1995 reported that patients given carnitine early in the course of their heart attacks who continued to take the supplement for one year afterward experienced significantly less "ballooning" of the heart muscle, which can cause heart failure. Another study done in the Philippines found that people given carnitine for eight weeks after a heart attack had less tissue damage—smaller regions of "dead" heart muscle—compared to people who did not receive the supplement.

Laboratory studies have found that carnitine helps keep the membranes of the red blood cells supple and flexible. The condition of the cell membranes is important because these cells must remain flexible in order to squish through the tiny openings of the capillaries. Some researchers speculate that carnitine may help to reduce heart tissue damage during a heart attack because it improves the condition of the cell membranes and thereby allows greater circulation.

Congestive heart failure. When the heart can no longer pump efficiently but has not stopped beating altogether, a person is said to be suffering from congestive heart failure. (For a more detailed description of this condition, see the section on congestive heart failure and CoQ10 on page 26.)

Carnitine has an outstanding record in assisting in the treatment of congestive heart failure. The results are so impressive that some experts believe that carnitine should be the treatment of choice when managing patients with this problem.

In one 1988 study, people with congestive heart failure were given 2 grams of carnitine a day. At the end of the study, their heart rates were lower, they had less fluid accumulation in the lungs and other tissues, and their breathing improved. The group taking carnitine was able to reduce their dependence on cardiac medications, and their cholesterol and triglyceride levels declined.

Arrhythmia. Arrhythmia is a condition in which the heart loses its regular rhythm and beats out of sync. Because the heart is not pumping efficiently, it may not receive a sufficient amount of blood. In fact, fully one-third of deaths due to cardiovascular disease are triggered by heart arrhythmias. Studies have found that carnitine can help to control arrhythmias.

Hypertension. High blood pressure, or hypertension, is more than a medical annoyance; it is one of the most accurate predictors of future cardiovascular disease, especially in people over age 65.

At the most basic level, hypertension refers to the pressure of the blood against the blood vessels as the heart pumps it through the arteries. A blood pressure reading consists of two numbers: the systolic pressure (the higher number, reflecting the pressure when the heart contracts) and the diastolic pressure (the lower number, re-

---

How High Is Too High?

Stage 1 hypertension: Systolic pressure of
                       140 to 159
                       Diastolic pressure of
                       90 to 99

Stage 2 hypertension: Systolic pressure of
                       160 to 179
                       Diastolic pressure of
                       100 to 109

Stage 3 hypertension: Systolic pressure of
                       180 to 209
                       Diastolic pressure of
                       110 to 119

Stage 4 hypertension: Systolic pressure of
                       210 or more
                       Diastolic pressure of
                       120 or more

flecting the pressure as the heart rests between beats). A normal blood pressure reading is 120/80, although the numbers fluctuate somewhat throughout the day. If your blood pressure is 140/90 or higher, you have hypertension and need to work on lowering it.

Hypertension cannot be cured, but it can be controlled. Untreated, high blood pressure can lead to stroke, heart disease and heart attack, loss of vision, and kidney failure because the heart must work harder than normal to pump blood. In fact, people with hypertension face a three times greater risk of heart attack and a seven times greater risk of stroke than those who have normal blood pressure.

High blood pressure is very common. Approximately 1 out of every 10 Americans suffers from hypertension. Those at increased risk include African Americans, people who smoke, those who are overweight, and those who have a family history of hypertension. High blood pressure also can be caused by arteriosclerosis (hardening of the arteries), atherosclerosis, congestive heart failure, kidney disease, diabetes, pregnancy, and hormonal disorders.

Hypertension is often called "the silent killer," because it strikes without warning. About 20 percent of Americans with high blood pressure don't know they have the condition, and only one-third have it under control.

Fortunately, most cases of high blood pressure can be lowered by diet and lifestyle changes. Carnitine also has been found to be effective at lowering blood pressure levels.

Warning Signs of Heart Disease

Some people learn they have heart disease when they experience the chest-crushing pain of angina. But many others don't receive any warning—until they have their first heart attack.

Heart attack victims often delay seeking medical help, frequently with fatal results. Most heart attack deaths occur in the first two hours, yet studies have found that many people wait four to six hours to get to an emergency room. Never ignore the warning signs of heart attack, including:

- Chest pain: an uncomfortable pressure, fullness, squeezing, or crushing feeling in the center of the chest that lasts two minutes or longer
- Severe pain that radiates to the shoulders, neck, arms, jaw, or top of the stomach
- Shortness of breath
- Paleness
- Sweating
- Rapid or irregular pulse
- Dizziness, fainting, or loss of consciousness

Not all of these warning signs occur in every heart attack. And some people, especially older people and diabetics, may not experience symptoms during a heart attack. (These so-called silent heart attacks can be detected only by an electrocardiogram.) If you suspect you may be experiencing a heart attack, get emergency medical help immediately. Doctors can prescribe a number of drugs that dissolve clots and reduce the oxygen demands on the heart, but these medications are more effective when given within one hour of the onset of a heart attack.

Carnitine and Cholesterol

High cholesterol levels have been implicated in the formation of cardiovascular disease. Carnitine helps to lower cholesterol levels by transporting the fats to the cells so that they can be burned for energy. Cholesterol—or serum lipids—burned within the mitochondria for the production of energy cannot accumulate in the cardiovascular system and cause plaque buildup.

Consider the findings of a 1983 study involving people who were given 1 gram of carnitine a day. The average total cholesterol levels were lowered from 295 to 234; at the same time, HDL levels increased and harmful triglyceride levels decreased.

Triglycerides are another type of blood fat that contains cholesterol. A study published in the journal *Circulation* found the risk of having a first heart attack was more than twice as high for those with the highest triglyceride levels as for those with the lowest levels. Desirable triglyceride levels are those under 200 milligrams per deciliter of blood. Cutting back on carbohydrates, particularly sugars and starches, may help to lower triglyceride levels. Numerous studies have shown that carnitine can help to reduce triglyceride levels, while raising helpful HDL levels.

How Do Your Cholesterol Numbers Add Up?

The evidence is undeniable: Study after study has shown that the higher your levels of blood cholesterol, the greater your chances of dying from heart disease. Fortunately, the converse is also true: For every 1 percent you lower your total cholesterol level, you reduce your heart disease risk by 2 to 3 percent.

To protect your heart, you need to find out your cholesterol levels and then figure out what all the numbers mean. Generally speaking, the lower your total cholesterol levels, the better. A level below 200 milligrams per deciliter would be ideal. There's more to the story, however.

Before cholesterol can enter the bloodstream,

it must attach itself to a lipoprotein. (Cholesterol is a fatlike substance, and blood is essentially water; the lipoprotein is necessary to transport the cholesterol through the blood, since fat and water don't mix.) There are two types of lipoproteins: low-density lipoproteins (LDLs) and high-density lipoproteins (HDLs). LDLs contribute to the formation of plaque deposits in the arteries, and HDLs help remove plaque deposits from the arteries.

Cardiovascular problems occur when the blood has too little HDL or too much LDL. To minimize your risk of cardiovascular disease, you want to have low levels of LDL cholesterol and high levels of HDL cholesterol.

You can raise your HDLs by exercising and eating a diet rich in fruits and vegetables. For postmenopausal women, estrogen replacement therapy also helps.

To lower your LDL levels, you must watch what you eat. The American Heart Association recommends limiting cholesterol intake to about 300 milligrams per day—the amount in one egg yolk. Restrict your daily fat intake to no more than 30 percent of calories from fat; only 10 percent of those should be from saturated fat. (That's 65 grams of fat and 22 grams of saturated fat for an average 2,000-calorie diet).

You also can lower your LDL levels by eating more soluble fiber. For example, studies have found that adding a bowl of oat cereal daily can lower LDL cholesterol by 5 to 10 percent.

Although cholesterol has a bad reputation for clogging the arteries, don't think of it as the enemy. Cholesterol is actually essential for a number of vital bodily processes, including nerve function, reproduction, and the formation of cell membranes. While cholesterol is found in some of the foods we eat, most of it is manufactured by the liver. In fact, each day our bodies churn out about 1,000 milligrams of the waxy white stuff, compared to the average dietary intake of about 325 milligrams for men or 220 milligrams for women.

Cholesterol presents problems only when the supply exceeds the body's demand for it. Unneeded cholesterol circulates in the bloodstream, where it can stick to the walls of the arteries and form the fatty deposits known as plaque. These cholesterol deposits build up over time and eventually restrict blood flow, causing cardiovascular disease. High cholesterol also has been implicated in causing gallstones, colon polyps, impotence, and high blood pressure. To avoid these problems, know your cholesterol levels and work to adjust them, if necessary.

Is Your Cholesterol Level Healthy?

	Desirable	Borderline	Undesirable
Total cholesterol	below 200	200–239	240 or higher
LDL cholesterol	below 130	130–159	160 or higher
HDL cholesterol	above 45	35–45	below 35
Ratio (total cholesterol/HDLs)	below 4.5	4.5–5.5	above 5.5

Lifestyle Changes to Protect Your Heart

Once cardiovascular disease is diagnosed, the goal of treatment is to halt—or even reverse—its progress. In addition to taking supplemental carnitine, there are some tried and true steps you can take to reduce your risk of heart disease:

- *Stop smoking.* Smoking constricts the arteries, raises blood pressure, increases arterial tearing, speeds atherosclerosis, and reduces oxygen levels in the blood. Smokers have two to four times the risk of heart attack as nonsmokers, and their heart attacks are more likely to be fatal. But there is hope: A decade after quitting, a former pack-a-day smoker has almost the same heart attack risk as if he or she had never smoked.

- *Exercise to keep your arteries strong and flexible*. Aerobic exercise helps prevent cardiovascular disease by lowering LDL cholesterol levels and raising HDL cholesterol levels, reducing blood pressure, keeping weight down, burning fat, lowering blood-sugar levels, and boosting relaxation. People who exercise regularly are about half as likely as sedentary people to have a heart attack. Furthermore, people who exercised as part of their rehabilitation after a heart attack had 25 percent fewer second attacks than people who didn't exercise.

- *Maintain a healthy body weight*. Excess body fat increases blood pressure and adds stress to the heart and circulatory system. People who maintain their ideal body weight are 35 to 55 percent less likely to have a heart attack than those who are obese (20 percent or more above their ideal weight).

- *Become more aware of your anger, anxiety, and fear*. These negative emotions trigger the release of adrenaline and increase blood pressure. These hormones also encourage the cells to release fat and cholesterol into the bloodstream. Defuse these emotions by practicing stress-management techniques.

- *Review all prescription and over-the-counter drugs with your doctor.* Some medications make your body retain more fluid, further straining your heart. Ask your doctor to assess the medications you're taking for possible adverse effects.
- *Know your history.* While there's nothing you can do to control your hereditary predisposition to cardiovascular disease, knowing your medical history can help you manage your risk factors. A family history of early heart attacks, high blood pressure, or stroke greatly increases your risk of developing cardiovascular disease. People whose parents or other close relatives have suffered a heart attack or stroke before age 55 should make a special effort to minimize their other risk factors.
- *Consume less caffeine.* Caffeine raises blood pressure temporarily and may have some long-term effects. According to a 1983 study published in the *American Journal of Cardiology*, coffee drinkers tend to have slightly higher blood pressure than people who don't drink coffee.
- *Limit salt intake.* Excessive consumption of salt (sodium chloride) makes it difficult for the kidneys to regulate blood pressure. High salt intake is especially difficult on the body when potassium and magnesium ingestion is low. High sodium relative to po-

tassium increases water retention and can elevate blood pressure. Strive to limit sodium intake to 1 to 2 grams per day.

- *Limit alcohol consumption.* While some researchers tout the cardiovascular benefits of modest drinking, consuming more than 30 milliliters of alcohol a day—an amount equal to 1 ounce of 100-proof whiskey, 8 ounces of wine, or two 12-ounce beers—can raise blood pressure.

Supplements for a Healthy Heart

What you eat and the dietary supplements you take can have a significant influence on the condition of your cardiovascular system. The following supplements have been found to be helpful in the treatment of heart disease.

- **Calcium**. Calcium is essential for blood clotting; it also plays a role in maintaining blood pressure. Take up to 1,500 milligrams a day.
- **Fiber**. A high-fiber diet helps lower cholesterol levels. The average American consumes only 11 grams of fiber a day, far short of the 25 grams experts recommend. If you don't care for high-fiber foods, take a psyllium-based supplement; follow package directions. One study found that people

who took one tablespoon of soluble-fiber supplement twice a day for eight weeks had a 7 percent reduction in their low-density lipoprotein (LDL) levels. Fiber tablets won't provide the same cholesterol-lowering benefits, since they contain a synthetic insoluble fiber.

- **Folic acid**. The body uses amino acids found in cow's milk and red meat to form homocysteine, an amino acid that helps create arterial lesions. Folic acid helps reduce homocysteine levels and lower the risk of heart disease. Take up to 400 milligrams a day.

- **Magnesium**. Magnesium is necessary to activate an enzyme that helps transport potassium to the cells. If the body lacks magnesium, and the potassium balance is disturbed, arrhythmias may result. Magnesium is also known to have relaxing and antispasmodic effects on the blood vessels. Some studies have found epidemiological evidence noting a link between low magnesium levels and deaths caused by cardiovascular disease. Many hospitals administer magnesium to patients when they are suffering from heart attacks or bouts of angina. Take up to 750 milligrams a day, or an amount equal to half your calcium supplement.

- **Niacin**. This vitamin, also known as vitamin B_3, plays an active role in more than 15 metabolic reactions, most of which are important in the release of energy from carbohydrates. Niacin lowers the "bad" LDL cholesterol and triglycerides while raising the levels of high-density lipoproteins (HDLs). It also improves circulation by dilating the blood vessels. Check with your doctor before taking niacin. Take up to 50 milligrams a day under your doctor's supervision. (At therapeutic doses, niacin can cause liver damage, so your doctor should conduct periodic blood tests to monitor your liver function.)

- **Potassium**. Potassium, which is found in the intracellular fluids in the body, helps maintain cell integrity and water balance. It is essential for muscle contraction and carbohydrate metabolism. Potassium is also an electrolyte and helps maintain the heart's electrical impulse and adequate heart rate. Take up to 5 grams a day.

- **Soy**. This protein contains two phytoestrogens—genistein and deidzen—that appear to help clear cholesterol from the blood. An analysis of 38 clinical trials found that people who ate an average of 47 grams of soy daily had a 13 percent drop in harmful LDL levels and a 9 percent drop in their total cholesterol. (Soy did not affect HDL levels.) Experts believe eating only 20 to 25 grams of soy daily—the equivalent of about 5 or

6 ounces of tofu—is enough to provide cholesterol-lowering benefits.

- **Vitamin A**. In addition to being powerful antioxidants, vitamin A and beta-carotene help to maintain elasticity in the tissues. Studies have shown that people who eat large amounts of beta-carotene have a significantly decreased mortality rate from cardiovascular disease compared with those who don't eat much beta-carotene. The vitamin A in a multivitamin supplement should be sufficient.

- **Vitamin C**. This vitamin is essential for cholesterol metabolism. It is responsible for the excretion of excess cholesterol from the body, and it helps the body balance "good" and "bad" lipids, one of the biggest factors in heart disease. Vitamin C also supports connective-tissue integrity within the vessel walls. Take up to 3,000 milligrams a day, in divided doses.

- **Vitamin E**. This antioxidant helps prevent free radical damage, in addition to helping the body maintain cardiac tissue and smooth muscle. It also keeps one particular form of LDL cholesterol from oxidizing and forming plaque deposits on the arteries. Vitamin E also inhibits the aggregation of platelets and inflammation inside vessel walls. Take 400 to 800 International Units a day.

Herbs for a Healthy Heart

In addition to carnitine, a number of herbs have a track record of helping with cardiovascular disease. The following herbs are available from health food stores; always follow package directions.

- **Dandelion** (*Taraxacum officinale*). This diuretic herb helps lower blood pressure and relieves chronic liver congestion. You can eat the fresh leaves in a salad or as a vegetable.
- **Garlic** (*Allium sativum*). This herb contains several sulfur compounds that block the biosynthesis of cholesterol. Garlic also helps expand the blood vessel walls by promoting their elasticity, increasing blood flow, and lowering blood pressure. Another chemical in garlic, ajoene, helps prevent blood clots. Use garlic liberally in cooking, or use a commercial preparation.
- **Ginkgo** (*Ginkgo biloba*). This herb helps dilate the blood vessels, reduce blood pressure, and improve overall circulation. Ginkgo flavonoids also act as antioxidants, reducing free radical damage. A number of studies have found ginkgo to be effective in

diseases that involve inadequate oxygen circulation to the tissues.

- **Hawthorn** (*Crataegus oxyacantha*). This quintessential "heart herb" enhances cardiac output in addition to opening up the peripheral vessels to improve overall circulation. It contains many chemical constituents that are known to strengthen the capillaries and vascular system. Studies have found that hawthorn can be effective in the treatment of high blood pressure, high cholesterol, angina pectoris, and atherosclerosis.
- **Motherwort** (*Leonurus cardiaca*). Small doses of this herb calm heart palpitations and normalize heart function.
- **Yarrow** (*Achillea millefolium*). This herb acts as a diuretic by dilating peripheral blood vessels. It helps lower blood pressure and reduces pressure on the heart.

For More Information

American Heart Association
7272 Greenville Avenue
Dallas, TX 75231
(214) 373-6300
www.americanheart.org

American Society of Hypertension
515 Madison Avenue, Suite 1212
New York, NY 10022
(212) 644-0650
www.ash-us.org

**Citizens for Public Action on Blood
Pressure and Cholesterol**
P.O. Box 30374
Bethesda, MD 20824
(301) 770-1711

International Atherosclerosis Society
6550 Fannin, No. 1423
Houston, TX 77030
(713) 790-4226
www.bcm.tmc.edu

Mended Hearts
7272 Greenville Avenue
Dallas, TX 75231-4966
(214) 706-1442
www.mendedhearts.org

National Heart Lung and Blood Institute
Information Center
National Institutes of Health
(301) 251-1222
www.nhlbi.nih.gov

National Heart Savers Association
9140 West Dodge Road
Omaha, NE 68114
(402) 398-1993
www.heartsavers.org

National Hypertension Association
324 East 30th Street
New York, NY 10016
(212) 889-3557
www.stepstn.com

SEVEN

Mental Sharpness: Carnitine and Brain Health

YOUR BRAIN IS AWASH IN CARNITINE. THE ACTUAL amount of carnitine in the brain, however, depends on the foods we eat, the nutritional supplements we take, the toxic exposures we tolerate, and our overall state of health. Over the years, the level of carnitine in the brain declines naturally, and not surprisingly, this loss of carnitine coincides with a loss in cognitive function. In addition, low levels of carnitine leave people more vulnerable to degenerative problems with the brain.

While nothing can be done to slow or stop the passage of time, taking carnitine supplements can go a long way toward minimizing the loss of brain function. Making wise lifestyle and nutrition choices can help to protect the brain. A number of human and animal studies have shown that carnitine can help stave off some of the mental decline associated with aging and can be very helpful in the treatment and prevention of some neurological diseases associated with aging.

Understanding Acetyl-L-Carnitine and Its Role in the Brain

Carnitine comes in two main forms: L-carnitine and acetyl-L-carnitine. (For details on the differences between carnitine and acetyl-L-carnitine, see page 8.) Both forms of carnitine are completely natural and nontoxic, but researchers have found that the brain responds best to the acetyl-L-carnitine form, probably because this form readily crosses the barriers and enters the brain.

While researchers do not fully understand how carnitine works, many believe the brain responds to acetyl-L-carnitine because its structure closely resembles that of acetylcholine, one of the most important neurotransmitters in the brain. Acetylcholine is one of the neurotransmitters responsible for memory and brain function. Many brain disorders, including Alzheimer's disease, involve defects in the brain's ability to produce and use acetylcholine. It appears that acetyl-L-carnitine functions much like the neurotransmitter acetylcholine in the brain; in other words, it helps the brain send and receive signals, making communication faster and more efficient among brain cells. By improving the function of the neurotransmitters, acetyl-L-carnitine restores some youthful vigor to the diseased or aging brain.

In addition, acetyl-L-carnitine works as an antioxidant, preventing free radical damage to the brain's cells. This is particularly important, since it is nearly impossible to replace brain cells when they die. And because carnitine in all its forms helps with energy production, acetyl-L-carnitine improves the metabolism or generation of energy within the cells of the brain.

Despite the many benefits to maintaining high levels of carnitine in the brain, the levels of acetyl-L-carnitine in the brain naturally drop off as we age. The levels begin to slip in midlife, which is why many experts recommend the use of acetyl-L-carnitine supplements beginning at age 40 to maintain optimal brain health.

Carnitine and Other Biochemical Changes in the Brain

In addition to promoting the neurotransmitters and acting as an antioxidant, acetyl-L-carnitine also performs several other highly specialized biochemical processes in the brain. Consider the following:

- Acetyl-L-carnitine helps to heal the brain by increasing levels of nerve growth factor, a compound found in the brain that helps protect the neurons.

- Acetyl-L-carnitine helps protect the myelin sheath that surrounds the nerves. The myelin sheath protects the nerves from damage and allows them to send and receive messages with great speed.

- Acetyl-L-carnitine protects the DNA and RNA in the cells. By protecting the cells' genetic material, acetyl-L-carnitine helps to protect the stability and integrity of the mitochondria within the cells.

- Acetyl-L-carnitine helps the brain use lipids as well as glucose for energy, according to a 1990 study published in the journal *Brain Research*. While the brain prefers to burn glucose, it can maintain a more stable energy supply if it can utilize alternative energy sources. The ability to use lipids for energy also protects the brain during bouts of low blood sugar.

A Word About Neurotransmitters

Neurotransmitters are chemicals found in the brain that allow brain cells or neurons to exchange signals and communicate using electrical pulses. Messages are passed along by chemical neurotransmitters that pass from one neuron to the next. Using this system, the brain's 50 billion neurons constantly trade information.

Acetyl-L-carnitine preserves brain function by protecting the receptors on the neurons that allow communication to take place. When the receptors are damaged—due to illness, trauma, free radical damage, or any other cause—the communication system breaks down. By defending the receptors from damage, acetyl-L-carnitine helps to facilitate communication among the neurons. The faster and more effectively the brain cells can communicate, the faster and more effective our brains work.

Research on Acetyl-L-Carnitine and the Brain

In the past decade or so, a number of studies have demonstrated the effectiveness of acetyl-L-carnitine in the treatment of Alzheimer's disease, Parkinson's disease, memory loss, depression, and mental functioning. The following section describes some of the key studies that have been done using acetyl-L-carnitine in the treatment of brain disorders.

Alzheimer's Disease. Some 4 million Americans—including two out of three nursing home patients—suffer from the debilitating effects of Alzheimer's disease and dementia. With Alzheimer's disease, the body malfunctions and gradually destroys the nerve cells in several key areas of the brain. As the disease progresses, the nerve fibers around the hippocampus—the brain's memory center—become crossed and knotted; these neurofibrillary tangles make it impossible to store or retrieve information. In addition to this internal short circuit, the brain also experiences a drop in the concentration of neurotransmitters, which further breaks down the body's communication network.

Alzheimer's disease is a type of dementia. The term "dementia" (or "senile dementia") refers to general mental deterioration, including memory loss, moodiness, irritability, personality changes, childish behavior, difficulty communicating, and an inability to concentrate.

Alzheimer's disease, dementia, or any other progressive loss of mental functioning shouldn't be considered a normal or inevitable part of the aging process. These conditions are signs that something has gone wrong. In a healthy person, intellectual performance can remain relatively uncompromised well into the 90s, provided the mind remains stimulated through learning. Most older people do not lose a significant amount of their mental functioning, and if they do, it is usually the result of a physical problem, such as a stroke.

Traditional medicine offers no effective treatments for Alzheimer's disease or dementia, but research done using acetyl-L-carnitine in the treatment of these conditions has been impressive. A comprehensive study done at the University of Pittsburgh School of Medicine involved giving Alzheimer's patients 3 grams of acetyl-L-carnitine a day for a year. Tests of cognitive function were given at the 6- and 12-month marks, and those study participants taking the acetyl-L-carnitine showed significantly less mental decline than those patients in the control group who did not take the supplement. In fact, those people taking acetyl-L-carnitine showed slower progression of the disease on 13 out of 14 parameters used to assess the condition. Both groups had started at roughly the same point of mental functioning, but the group taking acetyl-L-carnitine maintained their abilities while the others experienced a notable decline, according to the article published in 1995 in the journal *Neurobiology of Aging*. This finding is even more significant because the people taking acetyl-L-carnitine were older and presumably less responsive to treatment than those in the control group.

Other studies have found that acetyl-L-carnitine can be effective in treating cases of mental deterioration that are not severe enough to be classified as Alzheimer's disease. One double-blind, placebo-controlled study of 236 people with mild pre-Alzheimer's symptoms involved the use of 1,500 milligrams of acetyl-L-carnitine daily. The people receiving the supplement experienced significant improvement in memory and overall cognitive function.

Parkinson's Disease. Parkinson's is a paradoxical disease. When people suffer from it, some of their muscles become rigid and others contract involuntarily. People with Parkinson's disease may stoop, shuffle, and present a void, masklike, expressionless face while at the same time they suffer from an incessant tremor in the hands.

Parkinson's disease involves a failure of the body's internal communication system. When we are healthy, we take our bodies for granted, but every move we make, from kicking a ball to writing our names, requires thousands of coordinated communications between the brain, muscles, tendons, and bones. When these systems work well together, we think nothing of it, but when some part of the network breaks down, the effect can be devastating, as is the case with Parkinson's disease.

In 1817 British physician James Parkinson identified the disease that bears his name, although it was first called simply the shaking palsy. The disease, which afflicts more than 1 million Americans, involves damage to the middle section of the brain known as the *substantia nigra*, named for its blackish pigmentation. This midbrain area is the main supplier of dopamine, the neurotransmitter that allows for communication about movement between various parts of the body. When these cells die off and the dopamine supply dwindles, the nerve signals cross and muscle action goes haywire.

Parkinson's is a degenerative disease that usually first shows up when patients are in their 50s and 60s. There is no known cure for the disease, but the symptoms can be relieved through medication. Early treatment can help to slow the progression of the disease.

The cause of Parkinson's disease is unknown, although some experts suspect that a virus, malnutrition, or chemical exposure could be involved. Supporting evidence for the virus-trigger theory is that many people who survived the encephalitis epidemics between 1919 and 1926 (caused by a virus) developed Parkinson's years later. The toxin-trigger theory was bolstered by evidence of an outbreak of a Parkinson's-like disorder among drug addicts in San Francisco in the early 1980s.

In some cases, people develop symptoms of Parkinson's disease that actually prove to be side effects of medications. This is called Parkinson's syndrome rather than Parkinson's disease, and the symptoms disappear when the drugs are discontinued. If you suspect you have Parkinson's syndrome, review your use of all prescription and over-the-counter drugs, and discuss the issue with your doctor.

Recent animal studies have found that acetyl-L-carnitine can be helpful in slowing the progression of Parkinson's disease. Acetyl-L-carnitine is known to affect the production of dopamine in the brain, the very substance that is in short supply in Parkinson's patients. Acetyl-L-carnitine may protect the dopamine receptors in the brain and make them more responsive.

Memory Loss. Acetyl-L-carnitine is considered one of the most important "memory nutrients." According to researchers, acetyl-L-carnitine protects the memory receptors on the neurons. Studies have found that people taking 2 grams of acetyl-L-carnitine can focus their attention better and learn more efficiently than people in a control group not taking the supplements.

Depression and Mental Outlook. At some point in their lives, most people experience depression. Depression is not the same thing as sadness. While we all feel sadness in response to certain situations—the death of a loved one, the loss of a job, a divorce, or some other disappointment— depression is characterized by ongoing feelings of worthlessness, pessimism, sadness, and lack of interest in life. With clinical depression these feelings linger for weeks or months and ultimately become incapacitating.

Depression can be either a short-term, minor problem or a lifelong, life-threatening illness. Some people inherit a tendency to develop depression due to their brain chemistry. Other times the illness is brought on by physical conditions, such as stroke, hepatitis, chronic fatigue syndrome, chronic stress, thyroid disease, menopause, alcoholism, drug abuse—or even by the lack of natural light during the dark winter months. Some drugs, including over-the-counter antihistamines as well as many others, also can cause depression.

Whatever the cause, most cases of depression involve an imbalance of neurotransmitters, or chemical messengers, in the brain. While depression was once considered a shameful psychiatric condition, most experts now recognize that it usually has both physical and psychological triggers. It is an organic illness involving physical, biochemical changes in the body, so without help the person cannot "snap out of it," no matter how hard they try. While counseling and professional care can be crucial in recovery, taking acetyl-L-carnitine may also prove useful.

A number of studies have demonstrated that acetyl-L-carnitine can help to lift depression and mood disorders in older people. For example, one double-blind study using standard assessment scales for depression found that study participants who took 500 milligrams of acetyl-L-carnitine three times a day experienced significant relief from their depression. In fact, those who were most depressed were the ones who benefited most from treatment.

Warning Signs of Depression

It can be difficult to tell the difference between clinical depression and common sadness. But there are certain warning signs:

- Changes in sleep: either insomnia or sleepiness
- Changes in weight and eating habits: either weight gain or weight loss
- Loss of sexual desire or libido
- Chronic fatigue or tiredness
- Low self-esteem or self-worth
- Loss of productivity at work, home, or school
- Inability to concentrate or think clearly
- Withdrawal or isolation
- Loss of interest in activities that were once enjoyable
- Anger or irritability
- Trouble accepting praise or affirmation
- Feeling slow, every activity taking supreme effort

- Apprehension about the future
- Frequent weeping or sobbing
- Thoughts of suicide or death

These are all warning signs and diagnostic criteria for depression. If you or a loved one experiences three or more of these symptoms for two weeks or longer, contact a doctor or mental health professional for help. Don't try to treat serious depression by yourself. And if you or someone you're concerned about feels suicidal, immediately seek help from a specialist or a 24-hour hotline; look in the phone book under "Suicide Prevention."

Carnitine and Stress

Both physical and mental stress can be very damaging to the brain. When faced with stress, the body kicks in to the so-called fight-or-flight response, which involves a number of biochemical changes that happen in preparation for dealing with danger. In evolutionary terms, this high-intensity state made sense when quick bursts of energy were required to fight off predators or flee a dangerous situation. Of course, in our own daily lives we face fewer of these life-or-death threats, but the modern world remains full of stresses—financial worries, health concerns, deadline pressures, relationship problems. When confronted with these contemporary stresses, our bodies respond in much the same way as our prehistoric ancestors' once did.

Any stress in the body—either real or imagined—triggers an alarm in the hypothalamus in the midbrain. Then the autonomic, or involuntary, nervous system takes over. The hypothalamus shifts into overdrive, warning the body that it must prepare for an emergency. As a result, your heart races, your breathing speeds up, your muscles tense, your metabolism kicks into high gear, and your blood pressure soars. Your blood concentrates in your muscles, leaving your hands and feet cold and your muscles ready for action. Your senses become more acute: Your hearing becomes sharper, and your pupils dilate. You're ready to fight or flee.

As part of the intricate system of stress response, the adrenal glands on top of your kidneys begin to release adrenaline, epinephrine, cortisol, and other chemicals that inhibit the immune system and interfere with digestion, reproduction, growth, and tissue repair. While not harmful in short bursts, these stress responses can cause serious health problems if they continue for a long period of time. For example, someone working in a high-stress job or going through a difficult divorce might experience the physiological effects of stress for a prolonged period. Over the long haul, these stress responses can contribute to the development of disease. Chronic stress can elevate blood pressure, contributing to hypertension and cardiovascular disease; it can cause muscle tension, resulting in headaches and digestive disorders; it can suppress the immune system, leaving an individual prone to colds, flu, and a range of serious diseases. Mother Nature intended us to burn off these excessive stress hormones through physical activity, but most of us are forced to handle our stress sitting behind a desk or stuck inside a slow-moving car in a traffic jam.

Stress hormones can be brutal to the brain in particular. They can damage the neurons in the hippocampus, the part of the brain responsible for short-term memory. This is why short-term memory sometimes is inhibited in times of stress and why problems with short-term memory are one of the first signs of compromised mental functioning associated with aging.

As we age, our brains become less efficient at regulating levels of stress hormones because the receptors in the brain become less efficient at recognizing the presence of cortisol and other hormones. These receptors help the brain flip the "off" switch, telling the adrenal glands to stop producing hormones. If the receptors don't work well, the brain is exposed to higher levels of damaging stress hormones for longer periods of time. This process destroys the neurons and inhibits the production of neurotransmitters in the brain.

Fortunately, taking acetyl-L-carnitine can help the body manage stress and its physical manifestations. Studies have shown that acetyl-L-carnitine can help the body handle stress without experiencing a full-blown stress response. Specifically, acetyl-L-carnitine helps repair the cortisol receptors in the brain, allowing the brain to respond to stress hormones before their levels become excessive.

A number of studies support the use of acetyl-L-carnitine in the control of stress. A dramatic test done with laboratory mice demonstrates its effectiveness in assisting with stress management. Researchers placed mice into a maze with no escape. The mice were periodically exposed to a moderate electric shock—one strong enough to cause discomfort but not strong enough to cause significant pain. Within days the mice died, largely, the researchers speculated, because the situation was so stressful that the mice could not endure it either physically or emotionally.

In a second phase of the experiment, the researchers repeated the experiment, but they treated the mice with acetyl-L-carnitine prior to putting them in the maze. In this round of exposure to shocks in an escape-proof maze, all of the mice survived without any signs of impaired health. The researchers concluded that the carnitine helped the mice manage the stress and cope with their situation. While it is not fair to conclude from this type of animal experiment that acetyl-L-carnitine can protect humans from the ravages of stress, it does suggest that taking supplemental carnitine may provide some protective benefit that can help us manage stress with minimal physical problems.

Other Ways to Minimize Stress

While acetyl-L-carnitine can help to minimize the harmful effects of stress on the body, the practice of various stress-management techniques also can reduce daily stress. Studies have shown that people who practice relaxation exercises regularly are able to use mind-body techniques to lower their blood pressure and heart rate, alter their brain wave activity, reduce blood sugar levels, and ease muscle tension as well. Consider experimenting with the following techniques:

- **Biofeedback**. This technique involves training yourself to use your mind to voluntarily

control the body's internal systems. Almost
anyone can learn biofeedback, but it takes
practice.

- **Deep Breathing**. Deep breathing helps to
relax the body and quiet the mind. Unfortunately, most people don't breathe right
when stressed: Instead of inhaling deeply
and drawing in plenty of oxygen, they take
shallow, rapid, weak breaths, filling only
the top part of the lungs. This so-called
chest breathing, or thoracic breathing, fails
to oxygenate the blood adequately, making
it more difficult to manage stress.

- **Massage**. This technique offers a hands-on
way of reducing stress and promoting overall health. Massage—which involves the
soothing touch of the muscles, soft tissues,
and ligaments of the body—stimulates
blood circulation, slows the heart rate, and
lowers blood pressure.

- **Meditation**. Although it comes in many different forms or traditions, meditation basi-
cally involves focusing your complete
attention on one thing at a time. If you
haven't tried it, meditation can be harder
than it sounds: The mind tends to wander,
and maintaining concentration when faced
with a barrage of distracting thoughts can be
a real challenge. Meditation relieves stress
because it is impossible to feel tense or angry
when your mind is focused somewhere else.

- **Visualization**. You can use your imagination to relieve stress. Visualization—also known as guided imagery—builds on the idea that you are what you think you are; where the mind goes, the body will follow. If you think anxious thoughts, your muscles will grow tense; if you think sad thoughts, your brain biochemistry will change and you will become unhappy. If you think soothing, positive thoughts, you will relax and develop a more positive outlook.
- **Yoga**. This technique promotes relaxation while at the same time strengthening and stretching the muscles. It works to improve the functioning of the lymphatic system and reduce waste from muscle tension. Yoga, which involves deep breathing with systematic movement of the body in a series of postures or positions, can be good for preventing illness as well as for healing the system as a whole.

Think Smart: Other Supplements for Brain Protection

In addition to carnitine, daily doses of the following nutritional supplements have been found to be good for circulation and overall brain health:

- B complex vitamins (50 mg daily)
- Boron (3 mg daily)
- Flaxseed oil (1 tablespoon daily)
- Magnesium (400 mg daily)
- Omega-3 fatty acids (300 mg daily)
- Selenium (200 micrograms daily)
- Vitamin C (1,000 mg daily)
- Vitamin E (400 IU daily)
- Zinc (25 mg daily)

You also can keep your brain working its best by getting regular physical exercise; managing daily stress; avoiding the excessive use of alcohol, coffee, and stimulants; and giving your brain regular exercise by learning new skills and confronting mental challenges.

Some researchers believe that gluten-containing grains—such as wheat, oats, barley, and rye—can contribute to neurological disorders. Eliminate these grains from your diet at the first sign of a decline in mental functioning.

For More Information

Alzheimer's Disease

Alzheimer's Disease and Related Disorders Association
919 North Michigan Avenue,
Suite 1000
Chicago, IL 60611
(312) 335-8700
(800) 272-3900
www.alz.org

Alzheimer's Disease Society
2 West 45th Street, Room 1703
New York, NY 10036
(212) 719-4744
www.alzheimers.org

The American Journal of Alzheimer's Care and Related Disorders
470 Boston Post Road
Weston, MA 02193
(617) 899-2702

Parkinson's Disease

American Parkinson Disease Association
1250 Hyland Boulevard
Staten Island, NY 10305
(718) 981-8001
(800) 223-2732
www.the-health-pages.com/resources/apda

National Parkinson Foundation, Inc.
1501 Northwest 9th Avenue
Miami, FL 33136
(800) 327-4545
www.parkinson.org

Parkinson's Disease Foundation
William Black Medical Research Building
Columbia-Presbyterian Medical Center
650 West 168th Street
New York, NY 10032
(212) 923-4700
www.parkinsons-foundation.org

Parkinson Support Groups of America
11376 Cherry Hill Road, No. 204
Beltsville, MD 20705
(301) 937-1545

United Parkinson Foundation
833 West Washington Boulevard
Chicago, IL 60607
(312) 733-1893
www.pdf.org

Depression

**Depression and Related Affective
Disorders Association**
John Hopkins Hospital
600 North Wolfe Street
Baltimore, MD 21287
(410) 955-4647
www.med.jhu.edu/drada

**Depression Awareness, Recognition, and
Treatment (D/ART)**
National Institute of Mental Health
(800) 421-4211

**Depressives Anonymous: Recovering from
Depression**
329 East 62nd Street
New York, NY 10021
(212) 689-2600

Foundation for Depression and Manic Depression
24 East 81st Street, Suite 2B
New York, NY 10028
(212) 772-3400
www.fmd.org

National Depressive and Manic Depressive Association
730 North Franklin Street, Suite 501
Chicago, IL 60610
(312) 642-0049
(800) 826-3632
www.4woman.org

National Foundation for Depressive Illness
P.O. Box 2257
New York, NY 10116
(212) 268-4260
www.depression.org

National Mental Health Association
1021 Prince Street
Alexandria, VA 22314
(703) 684-7722
(800) 243-2525
www.nmha.org

Stress and Stress Reduction

Association for Applied Psychophysiology and Biofeedback
10200 West 44th Avenue, Suite 304
Wheat Ridge, CO 80033
(303) 422-8436
www.aapb.org

The Mind-Body Medical Institute
New Deaconess Hospital
Harvard Medical School
Boston, MA 02215
(617) 632-9530
www.mindbody.harvard.edu

The Stress Reduction Clinic
University of Massachusetts Medical Center
55 Lake Avenue North
Worcester, MA 01655
(508) 856-2656

EIGHT

Carnitine and Other Health Issues

CARNITINE MAY BE BEST KNOWN FOR ITS HEALING effects on the heart and brain—and its ability to increase energy, of course—but it has been found to improve a number of other conditions as well. Carnitine fortifies the body as a whole, allowing it to better handle the challenges of daily life and the stresses associated with illness, injury, and disease.

The Immune System

Carnitine owes much of its vast healing powers to its effect on the body's immune system, the system of defenses that protects the body from invasion by bacteria, viruses, and other pathogens. A strong immune system is essential to the maintenance of good health.

The challenge of the immune system is to allow the body to coexist with hundreds of millions of bacteria and other microorganisms but to remain on its toes, ready to attack and destroy any of those cells that threaten the body. Day and night the immune system hunts down renegade cells, unwanted invaders, and other potentially dangerous cells.

When the body's energy system fails to work its best—which happens when the body does not have enough carnitine—the immune system falters as well. During this energy crisis, the body spends its resources to meet the body's minimal needs, so little energy is left over to assist with the challenges of fighting viruses or healing the body after injury. When the immune system responds more slowly, some viral and bacterial agents have a chance to multiply and establish a foothold before the body's defenses gear up to stop them. The result: an infection that could be handled by a vigorous immune system could prove fatal to a weakened system.

Studies have found that carnitine helps to boost immune function by energizing the immune system and by acting as an antioxidant within the cells. In addition, researchers have found that carnitine actually can increase the number of immune cells available to come to your defenses.

Carnitine and Specific Health Problems

Earlier chapters described how carnitine helps in the treatment of fatigue, cardiovascular problems, and brain disorders; it also can be used in the treatment of a wide range of other conditions. The following sections describe those that respond well to carnitine supplementation.

Cancer

Every day our bodies produce more than 500 billion new cells. Every once in a while an error occurs, and our bodies form defective cells. This can be the beginning of cancer.

Cancer develops when oncogenes (the genes that control cell growth) are transformed by a carcinogen, or cancer-causing agent. In most cases the immune system identifies and destroys these aberrant cells before they multiply. But when the system breaks down, these fast-growing cancer cells reproduce, form a tumor, and invade healthy tissue. These tumors sap the body of nutrients and interfere with the tasks performed by the body's healthy tissue.

While cancer can develop at any age, it tends to affect older people more frequently, as they have been exposed to more carcinogens over a longer period of time. In many cases it takes years or decades for cancer-causing agents to do damage; other cancers grow and spread rapidly. Some experts speculate that older people may develop cancer more often because their immune systems become less proficient at detecting and destroying cancer cells.

While all cancers involve the uncontrolled growth of cells, the word "cancer" actually refers to more than 100 different diseases. Not all tumors are cancerous: Benign (noncancerous) tumors do not spread and infiltrate the surrounding tissue; malignant (cancerous) tumors do spread, or metastasize, through the blood vessels and lymph system to other areas of the body, where new tumors grow, Areas of the body where malignant tumors more commonly develop are the bone marrow, breasts, colon, liver, lungs, lymphatic system, ovaries, pancreas, prostate gland, skin, stomach, and uterus.

Cancer is the second most common cause of death in the United States, after heart disease. Despite its prevalence, the exact cause of cancer remains a mystery, although some experts argue that environmental factors—such as exposure to tobacco smoke, radiation, asbestos fibers, and toxic wastes—cause about 80 percent of all cancers. In addition, some people may inherit a greater sensitivity to carcinogens and thus a greater propensity to develop cancer.

While many types of cancer can be treated—especially if detected at the earliest stages—the disease varies greatly in its aggressiveness. Carnitine can help to bolster the body's defense mechanisms and restore its natural healing processes, but there is no "cure" that will work all the time. No single diet or program of supplements will work for all cancer patients, but carnitine can be an important supplement for most people with cancer because of its effects on the immune system. In addition, carnitine can help to support the body and provide energy to the cells during the course of chemotherapy, radiation, or surgery often used in the treatment of cancer.

Be on the Lookout

While many cancers grow undetected in the body for months, years, or decades before making themselves known, watch out for these common symptoms or warning signs of different types of cancer:

- A lump under the skin
- Persistent cough or chronic hoarseness
- Coughing up bloody sputum
- Difficulty swallowing
- Chronic indigestion
- A thickening or lump in the breast (usually in the outer or upper part of the breast); there may be dimpling or creasing of the skin near the lump
- Discharge from the nipple
- Bleeding or discharge, bleeding between menstrual periods

- Painful or heavy menstrual periods
- Obvious changes in bowel or bladder habits
- Blood in the stool or urine
- A persistent low-grade fever
- Headaches accompanied by visual disturbances
- Fatigue
- Excessive bruising
- Repeated nosebleeds
- Loss of appetite and weight loss
- Change in size or shape of the testes
- Persistent abdominal pain
- Continuous unexplained pain in the back or pelvis
- A sore or ulceration that does not heal
- A change in a wart or mole; pay special attention to the ABCD rule:
  - Asymmetry: Moles are symmetrical, cancers are not.
  - Borders: Moles have smooth borders: cancers have irregular or poorly defined borders.
  - Color: Variations in either shade or color from one area of the mole to another is a warning sign, as is the presence of red, white, or blue.

- Diameter: Moles larger than six millimeters (roughly the size of a pencil eraser) should be checked by a dermatologist.

For More Information

American Cancer Society
1599 Clifton Road, N.E.
Atlanta, GA 30329
(404) 320-3333
www.cancer.org

American Institute for Cancer Research
1759 R Street, N.W.
Washington, DC 20009
(202) 328-7744
www.healthfinder.gov

Cancer Care
1180 Avenue of the Americas
New York, NY 10036
(212) 221-3300
www.cancercare.org

Cancer Information Service
NCI/NIH
Building 31
9000 Rockville Pike
Bethesda, MD 20892
(800) 4-CANCER
www.cancer.gov

**National Coalition for Cancer
Survivorship**
1010 Wayne Avenue, 5th Floor
Silver Spring, MD 20910
(301) 650-8868
www.cansearch.org

People Against Cancer
604 East Street
P.O. Box 10
Otho, IA 50569-0010
(515) 972-4444
www.peopleagainstcancer.com

Diabetes

For diabetics, life is a balancing act. They must
carefully watch their blood-sugar levels: If the levels rise too high and stay there too long, they risk
damage to the nerves and blood vessels, which can
cause a number of health problems, including
blindness, infection, kidney problems, stroke, and
heart disease. But if blood-sugar levels drop too
low, even for a few minutes, they can become confused and even lose consciousness.

Normally the pancreas regulates this delicate
balance of sugar in the bloodstream. But the 14
million Americans with diabetes mellitus cannot
properly convert food (especially sugar) into en-

ergy, either because their bodies do not produce enough insulin (a hormone produced in the pancreas to regulate blood-sugar levels) or because their bodies don't properly use the insulin they do produce. Instead, diabetics must monitor their blood-sugar levels, adjusting their diet and exercise—or their oral medications and insulin injections—to meet these changing conditions.

There are two basic types of diabetes: the more severe form, known as Type I, insulin-dependent, or juvenile diabetes (about 15 percent of cases); and Type II, non–insulin-dependent, or adult-onset diabetes (about 85 percent of cases).

- Type I diabetes usually strikes sometime between the onset of puberty and age 30. It is caused by damage to the insulin-producing cells in the pancreas. For some reason it affects males more often than females.
- Type II diabetes usually occurs in middle-age and older people, especially those who are overweight. In most cases losing as little as 10 or 15 pounds helps control Type II diabetes. With Type II diabetes the pancreas produces insulin, but the sugar remains in the bloodstream. This more subtle version of the disease often goes undetected

until complications arise. Ultimately, up to 60 percent of Type II diabetics need supplemental insulin.

Both Type I and Type II diabetes seem to have a genetic component as well. Other possible causes include an immune response, following a viral infection, that destroys the cells in the pancreas. Diabetes also can follow other diseases, such as thyroid disorders, inflammation of the pancreas, or problems with the pituitary gland. About 5 percent of pregnant women develop diabetes, although the symptoms usually disappear after the baby is born.

Carnitine is a critical nutrient in the management of diabetes. Diabetics tend to have lower levels of carnitine in the blood and higher levels of carnitine secretion in their urine. Studies have found that carnitine helps insulin work more efficiently, so the body needs lower levels of insulin. For example, a 1999 study published in the *Journal of the American College of Nutrition* examined the effects of L-carnitine on insulin levels in Type II diabetics. The researchers found that in both diabetics and nondiabetics, carnitine significantly improved the body's ability to respond to insulin.

In addition, carnitine helps diabetics (and nondiabetics) lose weight. Maintaining a desirable weight is one of the most important ways for

Type II diabetics to control the disease. In fact, after losing excess fat, many Type II diabetics no longer need to take medications to lower their blood-sugar levels.

While carnitine is best known for assisting with fat metabolism, it also facilitates the burning of carbohydrates and helps prevent the loss of heart function that often occurs in people with diabetes.

As many as half of all diabetics develop neuropathy, or nerve damage, as a complication of the disease. Taking the acetyl-L-carnitine form of the supplement can help to prevent nerve damage.

As with other serious medical conditions, always discuss the use of carnitine supplements with your physician.

Is It Diabetes?

If you are overweight, over 40, or have a family history of diabetes, you might want to encourage your physician to test for diabetes at your annual physical. According to the National Institutes of Health, you may be diabetic if your blood glucose level is equal to or greater than 125 milligrams per deciliter (mg/dl) of blood first thing in the morning, or equal to or greater than 200 mg/dl two hours after consuming 75 grams of glucose, or if you experience hyperglycemia (a random glucose level of more than 200 mg/dl). A simple blood test for glucose levels can be performed at your doctor's office.

For More Information

American Diabetes Association
National Center
P.O. Box 25757
1660 Duke Street
Alexandria, VA 22314
(703) 549-1500
www.diabetes.org

Diabetes Research Institute Foundation
3440 Hollywood Boulevard, Suite 100
Hollywood, FL 33021
(305) 964-4040
www.drinet.org

International Diabetes Center
3800 Park Nicollet Boulevard
Minneapolis, MN 55416
(612) 927-3393
www.methodisthospital.com

Joslin Diabetes Center
One Joslin Place
Boston, MA 02215
(617) 732-2415
www.joslin.org

Gum Disease or Periodontal Disease

A beautiful smile requires not only beautiful teeth but healthy gums. Periodontal disease (literally meaning "disease around the tooth") is the major cause of tooth loss in older people. To some degree, periodontal disease affects up to 85 percent of the population. The older you are, the more likely you are to have the problem; more than half of all Americans over age 50 have signs of gum disease.

The gums that surround your teeth are called gingiva, and the network of gums, bones, and ligaments that form the tooth socket are called the periodontium. When you develop periodontal disease, you can experience swollen, bleeding, and receding gums as well as loose teeth.

Periodontal disease goes through three stages: gingivitis, periodontitis, and advanced periodontitis or pyorrhea. Stage 1 (gingivitis) refers to inflammation of the gums caused by plaque, the sticky bacterial film that forms on the teeth and gums. Plaque continuously builds up on the teeth, where it causes no harm as long as it is removed within 24 hours or so. After that time the plaque hardens into tartar (also known as calculus), which in turn produces toxins and enzymes that irritate the gums, causing them to become red and swollen. The gums also may bleed during brushing and flossing and begin to recede from the tooth.

If treated at this stage, periodontal disease can be controlled, since it has not yet damaged the bone and ligaments that hold the teeth in place. Untreated, however, the disease progresses to stage 2 (periodontitis) in which the plaque slips beneath the gums and begins to damage the roots of the teeth. Again, without proper treatment, the disease advances to stage 3 (advanced periodontitis or pyorrhea), which affects the bones and support system for the teeth. In stage 3, the gums often recede to the point that the teeth appear elongated; pockets form underneath the gums, where additional plaque and food can collect, causing bad breath and great gum irritation. The plaque and tartar under the gum line can cause infections that damage the bone, resulting in loose teeth and loss of teeth.

While inadequate tooth cleaning is the major cause of periodontal disease, other contributing factors include habitual cleaning and grinding of the teeth, mouth breathing, a high-sugar diet, and the use of tobacco, drugs, or alcohol. Hereditary, hormonal imbalances, and stress are other possible factors.

Carnitine helps to bolster the energy system, which can, in turn, help fight periodontal disease. Many Japanese dentists and periodontists recommend that their patients use carnitine and CoQ10 in the treatment of gum disease. Studies done in Japan have found that people with periodontal disease experienced marked improvement in their condition after taking carnitine and CoQ10 supplements for eight weeks.

For More Information

American Academy of Periodontology
737 North Michigan Avenue, Suite 800
Chicago, IL 60611-2615
(312) 787-5518
www.perio.org

American Board of Periodontology
Baltimore College of Dental Surgery
University of Maryland
666 West Baltimore Street
Baltimore, MD 21201
(410) 706-2432

American Dental Association
211 East Chicago Avenue
Chicago, IL 60611
(312) 440-2500
www.ada.org

National Dental Association
5506 Connecticut Avenue, NW, Suite 24
Washington, DC 20015
(202) 244-7555
www.natdent.org

HIV/AIDS Infection

Acquired immunodeficiency syndrome (AIDS) is a life-threatening disease characterized by the destruction of the body's immune system. AIDS is caused by infection with the human immunodeficiency virus (HIV). In most cases, the condition is recognized as a decrease in the ratio of T-helper to T-suppressor cells. The T-helper cells are lymphocytes (white blood cells) that help in the immune response against viruses and bacteria, and the T-suppressor cells are lymphocytes that suppress the immune response. This imbalance leaves the person with AIDS vulnerable to infections and cancer.

In the United States, the vast majority of cases involve people in high-risk groups—homosexual and bisexual men, intravenous drug users, hemophiliacs, people who have received blood transfusions or blood products, and heterosexuals having sexual contact with people in high-risk groups.

Because HIV and AIDS involves a weakening of the immune system, the immune-enhancing qualities of carnitine make it a helpful supplement. People with HIV and AIDS have low levels of carnitine, and studies have found that taking supplemental carnitine can strengthen the immune systems of people with HIV or AIDS in as little as 14 days. One study showed that carnitine is helpful in fighting cytomegalovirus infection, a common complication of AIDS.

Some of the drugs used to treat AIDS can deplete carnitine stores. For example, the drug AZT (zidovudine) has been found to lower carnitine levels in the body, making supplementation critical. Many experts recommend taking L-carnitine at levels of 1 to 3 grams a day, in divided doses. In addition, people with HIV and AIDS are often encouraged to take up to 1,500 milligrams of acetyl-L-carnitine to offer additional protection to the brain and nervous system.

For More Information

AIDS Action Council
1875 Connecticut Avenue, NW
Suite 700
Washington, DC 20009
(202) 986-1300
www.aidsaction.org

American Foundation for AIDS Research
120 Wall Street, 13th Floor
New York, NY 10005
(800) 39-AMFAR
www.foundationcenter.org

CDC National AIDS Clearinghouse
P.O. Box 6003
Rockville, MD 20849-6003
(800) 458-5231
www.cdcnpin.org

> **National Association of People with AIDS**
> 1413 K Street, N.W.
> Washington, DC 20005-3443
> (202) 898-0414
> www.napwa.org

Hypoglycemia

The brain depends on glucose (or sugar) for fuel. When the brain is starved for fuel because blood glucose levels drop too low, it responds by triggering a release of hormones designed to raise blood-sugar levels. These hormones can create the symptoms of hypoglycemia—sweating, tremors, rapid heart rate, anxiety, and hunger. When the onset of hypoglycemia is gradual, the symptoms may include dizziness, headache, cloudy vision, mental fogginess, emotional instability, and confusion.

Carnitine helps to minimize the wide swings in energy levels associated with hypoglycemia by helping the liver burn fat. As part of one study, medical students were put on a two-day fast; one group received carnitine supplements, while the other did not. The group receiving carnitine maintained normal blood-sugar levels, while the students who did not receive carnitine experienced blood-sugar levels associated with hypoglycemia.

Some researchers speculate that certain cases of

hypoglycemia may be caused by carnitine deficiency. Taking supplemental carnitine may help to prevent or control hypoglycemia and help the body maintain normal blood-sugar levels. For more information on hypoglycemia, see the resources on page 152 for diabetes, another condition involving irregularities in blood-sugar levels.

Infant Nutritional Support

When a baby is born, its body undergoes a dramatic shift in metabolism. In the uterus, the baby depended on a steady supply of glucose sent through the umbilical cord. After birth, the baby begins to burn long-chain fatty acids, which requires adequate levels of carnitine.

During pregnancy a mother needs to eat carnitine-rich foods since she must have adequate carnitine reserves to meet the baby's demands. Some obstetricians favor supplementing the mother's diet with carnitine in late pregnancy so that the baby will be well nourished at the time of delivery; this can be especially important to vegetarian women. If you are pregnant or nursing, discuss the matter of carnitine supplementation with your obstetrician.

After birth, infants need to receive carnitine, either through the mother's breast milk or through formula supplemented with carnitine. This additional carnitine is essential for babies' health because their livers cannot meet their carnitine demand. Even at 18 months, a child's liver can make only about 30 percent of the carnitine it will be able to make in adult life. Because of the importance of carnitine, it is regularly added to infant formula, especially soy formulas. (Cow's milk formula naturally contains some carnitine; soy formulas do not.)

For More Information

American Academy of Pediatrics
141 Northwest Point Boulevard
P.O. Box 927
Elk Grove Village, IL 60009-0927
(847) 228-5005
www.aap.org

American Pediatric Society
3400 Research Forest Drive, Suite B7
Spring, TX 77381-4259
(281) 296-0244
www.healthfinder.gov

Society for Developmental and Behavioral Pediatrics
19 Station Lane
Philadelphia, PA 19118-2939
(215) 248-9168
www.sdbp.org

Hypothyroidism

The thyroid gland regulates the metabolism, so an imbalance can affect almost all of the body's function. Symptoms range from mild to severe and life-threatening. Hypothyroidism involves the inadequate production of the thyroid hormones. In children, the symptoms include delayed growth and mental development. In adults, symptoms include low temperature, depression, difficulty losing weight, dry skin, headache, fatigue, menstrual problems in women, recurrent infections, and sensitivity to cold. Studies estimate that between 10 and 25 percent of the population may experience thyroid problems.

People with hypothyroidism often have low levels of carnitine, but the condition responds well to supplementation. In addition, people with hypothyroidism often have high levels of fat in their blood, another problem that can be helped with carnitine supplementation. There is no apparent link between carnitine and hyperthyroidism or excessive production of thyroid hormones.

For More Information

Thyroid Foundation of America
Ruth Sleeper Hall
RSL 350
40 Parkman Street
Boston, MA 02114-2698
(617) 726-8500

Infertility (Male)

Most couples who want to have children are successful—some sooner, some later. Typically, half of the couples who decide to stop using contraception will conceive within three to five months, and about 85 percent of the couples will conceive within a year. However, that leaves 15 percent—or roughly one out of every six couples—who will experience fertility problems.

Impaired fertility has many causes. For about 35 to 40 percent of couples, the problem lies with the woman; for another 35 to 40 percent, the problem lies with the man; and in the rest, both partners have a problem or the cause is unknown.

Among men, abnormal sperm—either low sperm count or inferior sperm quality—is to blame for most fertility problems. It may take only one sperm to fertilize an egg, but the average ejaculation contains between 40 million and 150 million sperm. Most of these sperm don't stand a fighting chance of getting within striking distance of the awaiting egg; some 80 to 90 percent of them are killed off by vaginal fluids. Due to this intense screening process, men who ejaculate fewer than 60 million sperm may have difficulty impregnating their partners. In medical terminology, oligospermia means low sperm count and azoospermia means the absence of living sperm in the semen.

Not surprisingly, the number of sperm in an ejaculate and the degree of fertility are strongly correlated. But even men with low sperm counts can impregnate their partners. In fact, studies at fertility clinics have found that 52 percent of men whose sperm counts were below 10 million per milliliter of ejaculate achieved pregnancy, as did 40 percent of those with sperm counts as low as 5 million per milliliter of ejaculate.

Numbers count, but when it comes to fertility, sperm quality is even more important than quantity. A man can have a high number of sperm, but if a majority of them are abnormally shaped or poor swimmers, he can have a harder time becoming a father than a man with fewer sperm of a higher quality. Sperm quality is based on several factors, including motility (how fast and straight the sperm swims) and morphology (sperm size and shape). At least 60 percent of the sperm should be normal in appearance and motility.

Problems with sperm can stem from a number of causes, including varicocele (a varicose vein in the scrotum), prostate infections, duct obstructions, ejaculatory dysfunction, mumps, alcohol use, nicotine use, illness, or excessive fatigue.

Studies have found that taking supplemental carnitine can improve sperm quality and motility. As part of a study conducted in Italy, one hundred men were given 3 grams of L-carnitine daily, in divided doses. When assessments of their sperm were done at two, four, and six months, the researchers noted a statistically significant increase in sperm quantity and quality.

Carnitine also helps to protect fertility by helping the body manage stress. Stress can interfere with fertility by upsetting the delicate hormonal balance required for reproduction.

For More Information

American College of Obstetricians and Gynecologists
P.O. Box 96920
409 Twelfth Street, S.W.
Washington, DC 20090-6920
(202) 638-5577
www.acog.org

American Self-Help Clearinghouse
Northwest Convenant
25 Pocono Road
Denville, NJ 07834
(201) 625-7101
www.mentalhelp.net

American Society for Reproductive Medicine
1209 Montgomery Highway
Birmingham, AL 35216-2809
(205) 978-5000
www.asrm.org

Fertility Resource Foundation
877 Park Avenue
New York, NY 10021
(212) 744-5500

RESOLVE, Inc.
1310 Broadway
Somerville, MA 02144-1779
(617) 623-0744
www.resolve.org

PMS

Premenstrual syndrome (PMS) is a very real problem that challenges many women every month. More than 150 different symptoms have been associated with PMS, but the most common include breast tenderness, fatigue, bloating and weight gain, food cravings, anger, depression, and irritability. PMS occurs between ovulation and the start of the menstrual cycle, or about two weeks before monthly bleeding begins. Many women suffer from PMS in silence, ashamed and embarrassed to talk about their feelings.

PMS is not a disease; it is a natural consequence of the hormonal changes that occur during the menstrual cycle. Carnitine can help minimize the symptoms of PMS by regulating the energy system.

Carnitine helps maintain hormonal balance by promoting the health of the pituitary gland and hypothalamus in the brain. Because the hormone system is regulated by the brain, acetyl-L-carnitine is the preferred form of carnitine for the regulation of PMS.

As part of the PMS response, some women overeat to maintain their energy levels. Carnitine can help to keep blood-sugar levels even, which can minimize food cravings and help control binge eating.

For More Information

National Women's Health Resource Center
2425 L Street, NW
Washington, DC 20037
(202) 293-6045
www.healthfinder.gov

Society for Menstrual Cycle Research
1059 North 104th Place
Scottsdale, AZ 85258
(480) 451-9731

Stroke

A stroke is like a heart attack in the brain. Just as part of the heart dies when deprived of oxygen during a heart attack, so a part of the brain dies when deprived of oxygen during a stroke. A thrombotic stroke occurs when an artery in the brain is blocked by a clot or by atherosclerosis; an embolic stroke occurs when a small clot (known as an embolus) forms elsewhere in the body and moves to the brain, where it lodges in an artery and blocks the flow of blood. Hemorrhagic stroke occurs when an artery ruptures, usually due to high blood pressure. While hemorrhagic strokes are less common—only about 20 percent of all strokes—they are much more lethal, causing about 50 percent of all stroke-related deaths.

In the aftermath of a stroke, the person loses the bodily functions associated with the part of the brain that was destroyed. Symptoms of a stroke include slurred speech or loss of speech; sudden severe headache; double vision or blindness; sudden weakness or loss of sensation in the limbs, or loss of consciousness. These symptoms can occur over a period of a few minutes or hours, and they can occur on one side of the body or both.

Stroke is the nation's third leading cause of death and the leading cause of adult disability. Experts estimate that as many as 80 percent of all strokes can be prevented, either through changes in lifestyle or through the use of drugs to control high blood pressure and the tendency to form blood clots.

The use of acetyl-L-carnitine can help in the recovery from stroke. According to a 1997 study reported in the *Annals of Emergency Medicine*, treatment with acetyl-L-carnitine can minimize neurological damage following a stroke, provided the supplementation is administered promptly.

For more information on stroke, see the resources for cardiovascular disease on page 112–13.

Surgery

Carnitine can be a very important supplement to take to strengthen the body before surgery. When the body has optimal nutrition prior to surgery, it has the resources to speed healing, reduce tissue scarring, and reduce the risk of complications.

Carnitine and CoQ10 help to minimize free radical damage, which can be especially important during heart surgery. Studies have found that taking 1 gram of carnitine daily in the three or four days before surgery can help the heart survive surgery without complications.

In addition, taking supplemental acetyl-L-carnitine helps prevent damage to the brain during major surgery. When the body undergoes general anesthesia, the brain sometimes experiences periods of oxygen deprivation. The acetyl-L-carnitine protects the brain from the memory loss and damage to brain tissue that can result from these times without oxygen.

Other essential nutrients that promote the growth and healing of tissues include vitamin A, vitamin C, and zinc. Always consult your surgeon before taking supplements to encourage wound healing.

For More Information

American Academy of Wound Management
1720 Kennedy Causeway, Suite 109
North Bay Village, FL 33141
(305) 866-9592
www.aawm.org

American Board of Surgery
1617 John F. Kennedy Boulevard, Suite 860
Philadelphia, PA 19103
(215) 568-4000
www.absurgery.org

Injury Control Research Center
Harvard University
School of Public Health
718 Huntington Avenue, 2nd Floor
Boston, MA 02115
(617) 432-2123
www.injurycontrol.com

NINE

The Safe and Effective Use of Carnitine

AFTER READING THE PREVIOUS CHAPTERS, YOU know that carnitine can help many people maximize their energy, optimize their athletic performance, and burn fat to keep their weight under control. You also know that carnitine can improve cardiovascular health and improve brain metabolism, and that this simple nutrient can have a significant effect on the treatment of other illnesses and medical conditions. You know that carnitine offers these significant benefits without the threatening negative side effects common with many prescription drugs used to achieve these same goals.

Thousands of Americans enjoy the benefits of carnitine supplements. Despite the supplement's impressive record, keep in mind that carnitine is not a miracle drug; the medical problems described in this book are complex and multifaceted. While carnitine may play an important role in your treatment and overall health regimen, you should not self-medicate when seeking treatment for health problems. *Once again, be sure to discuss your overall treatment plan and the role of carnitine in your healthcare with your doctor or other health professional.*

In addition, if you are currently taking any prescription drugs, do not discontinue your treatment or medication without discussing the matter with your doctor. Because carnitine can be very effective at promoting energy and weight loss, strengthening the heart, and improving brain function, you may find that you no longer need the same dosages of prescription medications to deal with these problems. This is a matter that should be managed by your physician. Stopping or changing your existing medication routine can put you at risk of developing serious physical and emotional symptoms, depending on the medication you are taking.

Is Carnitine Right for You?

The evidence presented earlier in this book demonstrates that carnitine can provide life-transforming changes in many people. However, like almost any other drug or nutritional supplement, carnitine is not right for everyone. Most physicians do not recommend the use of carnitine for people with the following medical conditions:

- Epilepsy or other seizure disorders
- Manic depression (also known as bipolar depression)
- Impaired renal (kidney) function

NOTE: *If you would like to take carnitine supplements but you have a seizure disorder, manic depression, or kidney problems, discuss the matter with your doctor before taking any supplements.*

Understanding Carnitine and CoQ10

Many people use carnitine and CoQ10 to improve their health. The following questions can help to answer some common questions about the use of carnitine and CoQ10.

Q: How much carnitine should a person take?

A: Most experts recommend a daily dosage of carnitine ranging from 1,000 to 3,000 milligrams a day in divided doses. They suggest starting with a dose of 500 mg with breakfast and 500 mg with lunch. People who need to increase the dosage may add a third 500-mg dose with dinner.

Some healthcare professionals recommend taking up to 3,000 mg per day by taking 1,000 mg of carnitine with each meal. It is best to start with the lower dose; increase the amount of carnitine you take gradually, and only if you notice an improvement on the higher dosage.

Keep in mind that the recommended dosage does not vary with the condition being treated. In other words, experts recommend the same dosage whether the supplement is used to boost energy or strengthen the heart.

NOTE: *People undergoing hemodialysis (dialysis of the blood) should avoid higher doses of carnitine; some people undergoing this treatment have had problems with their triglyceride levels and with platelet aggregation (the formation of blood clots) when taking carnitine at higher doses (3 grams per day or higher). Carnitine supplementation should be safe at lower levels; discuss the matter with your doctor.*

Q: How much CoQ10 should a person take?

A: As with carnitine, experts recommend that people begin with a low dose of CoQ10 and increase it as needed. Doctors suggest that most people start by taking 30 mg of CoQ10 with breakfast and with lunch. Those people who do not respond may add a third dose of carnitine with dinner, they may add a third 30 mg dose of CoQ10 as well.

Experts recommend those people who increase their dose of carnitine to 1,000 mg at mealtimes should increase their CoQ10 dose to 60 mg as well. Remember that carnitine and CoQ10 appear to work synergistically when combined; the dose of CoQ10 should be increased in proportion to the dose of carnitine.

Q: What side effects should I look for?

A: Carnitine has never been found to cause an overdose or a toxic response in any human clinical trial, according to the *Physician's Desk Reference*. In fact, it is considered so safe that it is added to infant formula. According to research done on adults, some people do report, however, that they have more vivid dreams at night when taking carnitine. (This side effect was reversible; the dreams ceased when the level of carnitine supplementation was reduced.) Some people enjoy vibrant dreams, others do not.

Q: Should carnitine and CoQ10 be taken with water?

A: Yes, always. Experts recommend that people drink a full glass of water after tak-

Bottoms Up

Most people experience an ongoing state of physical drought: They don't drink nearly enough water to meet their body's needs. The body needs water to wash away toxins and speed their elimination. How much water is enough? Take your weight in pounds and divide that number in half—that total is the ideal number of ounces of water you should drink each day. For example, if you weigh 150 pounds, you should consume 75 ounces of water each day.

Drink a small amount of water with meals—about 4 to 6 ounces. This is enough to aid digestion, but not so much that you dilute hydrochloric acid, which is needed for the digestion of protein. Drink most of your fluids a half hour before meals and between meals.

The best water has been filtered by reverse osmosis. (You can buy a reverse-osmosis unit, which filters water as it is pumped from the faucet, for about $500 to $1,000.) Don't drink distilled water, since its lack of minerals can draw other minerals from the body, leaving your system out of balance. Instead, drink filtered or purified water.

ing the supplements at each meal. The water helps with the absorption of the nutrients. In addition, water plays a number of other essential roles in the body, and most people don't drink enough water every day.

Q: Where can I find carnitine and CoQ10 supplements?

A: Carnitine and CoQ10 supplements are available in drugstores, health food stores, supermarkets, discount department stores, and on the Internet. You may have to hunt around a bit to track down carnitine; some stores put it on the same shelf as the amino acids, while others stock it with the vitamins or nutritional supplements. CoQ10 may be placed with vitamins or with the section on nutritional enzymes. If you have any trouble locating either carnitine or CoQ10 in a store, ask for help. Both supplements are quite popular, so they should be available in a well-stocked store.

Q: If a person skips a meal, is it safe to take carnitine and CoQ10 supplements?

A: Experts recommend that people avoid taking either supplement on an empty stomach. Some people find the supplements can cause nausea if taken without food and water. The food and water help the body absorb the nutrients, and they also help to buffer the stomach.

Q: Should a person make up a missing dose if he or she forgets to take the supplements during a meal or even for an entire day?

A: No, experts do not recommend taking additional supplements if a person skips a dose. People should try to be diligent about taking the supplements since they need to take the supplements regularly to enjoy their health-promoting effects.

Q: Can a person take carnitine and CoQ10 in combination with other prescription or over-the-counter medications?

A: There are no known adverse drug interactions between carnitine or CoQ10 and other drugs or nutrients. However, if you are taking any medications, check with your doctor before taking carnitine, CoQ10, or any other nutritional supplement. It's always better to err on the side of caution when it comes to protecting your health.

Q: Carnitine is available as both L-carnitine and acetyl-L-carnitine. Which type of carnitine is best?

A: It depends on a person's reason for taking carnitine. Most carnitine is sold as either L-carnitine or acetyl-L-carnitine; both can be used safely and effectively to improve overall health.

In the body, L-carnitine is broken down into acetyl-L-carnitine. In technical terms, the L-carnitine is converted into an acetyl ester of L-carnitine. Both L-carnitine and acetyl-L-carnitine help to shuttle fatty acids into the cells' mitochondria to produce energy. L-carnitine has proven particularly efficient at energizing the heart muscle. Acetyl-L-carnitine has been found to help perform certain metabolic functions in the brain, making it a superior choice when carnitine is taken for issues involving brain metabolism.

The type of carnitine a person should take depends on the reason for choosing the supplement. Experts use the following guidelines when recommending carnitine:

- For weight loss, use either L-carnitine or acetyl-L-carnitine.
- For energy enhancement, use either L-carnitine or acetyl-L-carnitine.
- For heart strengthening and cardiovascular benefits, use L-carnitine.
- For support of brain metabolism and other cerebral and nerve functions, use acetyl-L-carnitine.

People who want to enjoy the benefits of both L-carnitine and acetyl-L-carnitine can use the products in combination. In fact, some experts believe there may be a synergy or combined benefit by using both L-forms of carnitine together. When using both types of carnitine, do not double your total dosage; instead, divide each dose between L-carnitine and acetyl-L-carnitine.

Q: What is D-carnitine? Is it a substitute for L-carnitine?

A: No. *Always use L-carnitine*. The D-form actually interferes with the body's use of the L-form of carnitine. In fact, a number of studies have found that the D-form and the D,L-form of carnitine can cause health problems associated with carnitine deficiency. For example, studies have shown that people taking D,L-carnitine may experience severe muscle fatigue and a dangerous reduction in their exercise tolerance, while those taking the recommended L-carnitine experience strengthening of the heart and skeletal muscles. The bottom line: *Do not take D-carnitine or D,L-carnitine.*

Q: How much does carnitine cost?

A: A month's supply of carnitine costs about $60, depending on the amount you take. Some chain stores or mail-order houses offer sales or two-for-one offers periodically. Shop around and compare prices to find the best value for your money.

Q: Is carnitine covered by insurance?

A: Not for most people. Carnitine is available by prescription under the brand name Carnitor, and the U.S. Food and Drug Administration has approved it for the treatment of specific carnitine deficiency diseases, rare conditions that primarily affect children. Carnitine is one of very few nutritional supplements that has undergone the rigorous testing required by the Food and Drug Administration for drug approval.

Carnitine may be covered by your insurance if it is prescribed by your doctor (depending on your specific health insurance coverage), but over-the-counter supplements are not, even if your doctor approves of your carnitine routine. If you can afford to take carnitine, most experts consider the health benefits worth the cost of the supplements. Carnitine is usually sold in 250-, 400-, or 500-milligram capsules. It is also available in pill and liquid forms.

Q: What form of CoQ10 should a person take?

A: Most experts recommend CoQ10 in micronized, water-soluble soft gel capsules because these can be more easily absorbed by the body than CoQ10 in hard capsule form. CoQ10 is sold in 15-, 30-, 60-, 75-, and 100-milligram soft gels and capsules.

Q: How can you be sure the carnitine and

CoQ10 supplements are responsible for the changes in your health?

A: It can be very difficult for a person to determine whether changes in energy level and health can be attributed to a carnitine and CoQ10 supplement program and which may be caused by an improved outlook or other factors. One way for a person to monitor his or her progress is to keep a health diary of the first three or four weeks of supplement use. If you would like to keep a health diary, take a couple of minutes every few hours to jot down a few notes about how you feel. Record the foods you eat, the number of hours you sleep, your mood, your energy level, your exercise habits, and other applicable measures of your physical condition. Don't record more information than necessary; if you make the task too onerous, you may not keep up with it for long.

Over a period of several days or weeks, you may begin to recognize a change in patterns. On days you feel dynamic and energetic, look at the factors that might have supported those changes. Likewise, when you feel tired or depressed, review the foods you ate or the amount of exercise you got and look for links between your health habits and your physical state.

A journal can be particularly helpful in

deciding whether you need to increase your dosage of carnitine and CoQ10. You should recognize improvements in your mood and energy level that coincide with the amount taken of each supplement.

Q: How long should a person take carnitine?

A: According to experts, carnitine can be taken on an ongoing basis without adverse health effects. Some people who use carnitine as part of a weight-loss program stop using it when they reach their target weight, but many others continue taking the supplement because they enjoy its other health benefits.

Beyond Carnitine Supplements

While carnitine can go a long way toward promoting your health and energizing your body, you can't expect simply to swallow a capsule and transform your life. In fact, your carnitine program also includes three important changes in lifestyle—you need to eat a mitochondria-friendly diet, get sufficient exercise to encourage the production of energy, and sleep long enough and well enough to give your body a chance to heal and rejuvenate itself. The rest of this chapter covers these three critical components of overall health.

The Importance of Diet:
Eating Mitochondria-Friendly Foods

Food is fuel. Although many people become very emotionally involved in the decisions they make about the foods they eat, the body processes every bite of food we eat in the same way. Whether we dine on cheeseburgers and fries or fresh fruits and veggies, our bodies break down the food into one of three basic substances: glucose (simple sugars), amino acids (the building blocks of protein), or fatty acids (the building blocks of fats). Only after foods have been divided into these categories can our bodies use the nutrients for the production of energy and for other metabolic processes.

Ideally, you should consume a diet rich in mitochondria-friendly foods that can be easily broken down into the necessary nutrients. The following nutritional tips can help you make wise food choices to help your body efficiently utilize its nutrients.

- *Avoid processed foods.* Our bodies use digestive enzymes to break down a food into its nutritional components. Unfortunately, many processed foods contain preservatives and chemicals that our body's enzyme system cannot handle. Our bodies waste a lot of energy and are exposed to significant levels of toxins by trying to break down these foreign substances. The buildup of these toxins can damage the mitochondria, which inhibits energy production in the cell and makes it even more difficult for the cell to handle the processed foods. Instead of eating processed foods, choose whole, natural foods. Read food labels and steer clear of foods containing preservatives whenever possible.

- *Don't overeat.* Overeating leaves you feeling uncomfortable and puts a great deal of stress on your entire body. Your energy-producing mitochondria can become fatigued by working so hard to handle all the food you have consumed either at a given meal or during the day. In addition to limiting the size of your meals so that you don't feel bloated, some experts recommend limiting your food intake to a 12-hour period. For example, you might eat breakfast at 7 A.M. and your final meal of the day at 7 P.M. Following this regimen provides your body with a much-needed period of digestive rest.

- *Avoid refined sugars.* Sugar in general and refined sugar in particular can cause the body to enter into an unhealthy rollercoaster of food cravings. When you eat foods high in sugar, the body converts the sugar into glucose, triggering a rapid increase in blood-sugar levels. In turn, the body experiences a short-lived surge of energy. The brain responds to the high blood-sugar levels, however, by telling the pancreas to release insulin, the hormone that helps the body use sugar. The insulin rush causes the body to feel sluggish and weak again—and it fuels a craving for the very sugars that created the problem in the first place. Refined sugars are found in candies, cakes, sodas, sweetened cereals, white rice, and some breads. To avoid the wild ride, avoid refined sugars whenever possible. Carnitine can help you avoid the feelings of fatigue that promote the sugar-abuse cycle.

- *Pace your eating throughout the day.* To reinforce your body's circadian rhythms and digestive cycles, try to eat on a regular schedule. Our bodies release certain digestive hormones at fixed intervals; erratic eating patterns can interfere with the regularity of your body's hormonal cycles.
  - —Strive to start the day with a well-balanced breakfast that provides nutrients and energy for the day's activities. People who eat breakfast are less likely to overindulge at lunch. If you can't stomach an early breakfast, at least have a healthful midmorning snack.
  - —Eat lunch near noon, not in the middle

of the afternoon. If you wait until you feel famished to eat, you're much more likely to feel fatigued and to overeat. Also, eating a late lunch can push the dinner hour back to the point that you go to bed with a full stomach. If you tend to experience a period of low energy in the afternoon, be sure your lunch includes plenty of protein and not too much starch. And, of course, forgo the sugary desserts and snacks that can trigger a sluggish feeling in the afternoon.

—Eat dinner at least two hours before you plan to go to bed. You don't want to go to sleep with a stomach full of food that needs to be digested.

- *Consume fats wisely.* Many people, particularly those concerned about weight loss, worry about consuming too much dietary fat. In truth, our bodies need some fat; ultra–low-fat diets can cause weakness because our bodies must work hard to release fatty acids from muscle tissue or stored fat. Fats also are needed for growth, hormone production, and other essential body processes. They carry and store the fat-soluble vitamins (vitamins A, D, E, and K). On a cosmetic level, inadequate dietary fat can lead to dry skin and lackluster hair; and, on a sensual level, fat adds flavor to food, making the very act of eating more pleasurable.

(You don't need to deny yourself pleasure in order to lose weight.)

Too much fat is, of course, unhealthy. The typical American consumes about 40 percent of calories from fat, despite warnings that fat intake should be limited to 30 percent of calories. To achieve the 30 percent goal, people who consume 1,800 to 2,400 calories per day should consume 60 to 80 grams of fat. One gram of fat has 9 calories; one gram of protein or carbohydrate has 4 calories. The body needs about 10 percent of its calories from fat (about 20 grams a day) to perform its necessary functions.

In addition to watching total fat, you also must keep an eye out for the *type* of fat you consume. Dietary fats consist of combinations of three types of fatty acids—saturated, polyunsaturated, and monounsaturated:

- —Saturated fats tend to be hard at room temperature.

  Examples: Butter, cheese, chocolate, coconut oil, egg yolk, lard, meat, palm oil, vegetable shortening.
- —Polyunsaturated fats tend to be liquid at room temperature.

  Examples: Corn, cottonseed, fish, safflower, soybean, and sunflower oils.
- —Monounsaturated fats fall in between.

Examples: Avocados; canola, cashew, olive, and peanut oils.

- *Avoid low-calorie diets for weight loss.* Instead of cutting calories to lose weight, eat mitochondria-friendly foods to increase energy and you won't feel the need to eat as much. Many dieters assume that low-calorie diets will cause the body to break down fat for energy, but this is not the case. Instead, the body finds it much more efficient to break down protein for energy before turning to fat. When the diet does not contain enough calories, the body consumes its own protein (typically in the form of muscle fiber), causing the dieter to feel weak and worn down. The most efficient way to lose weight is to consume mitochondria-friendly whole foods and to get plenty of exercise. This strategy leaves the body feeling energetic and healthy—and it results in weight loss as well.
- *Choose organic foods.* Whenever possible, buy fruits, vegetables, and meats that are certified organic. Organic foods should have less pesticide residue than nonorganic products. Look for the U.S. Department of Agriculture's organic label, which recently replaced the private certification network that was in place before 1998.
- *Don't cook in the microwave.* While you can use the microwave to heat water for tea,

avoid using it to prepare food. Microwave ovens heat the food to such a high temperature that the proteins coagulate, thus diminishing the nutritional value of what you're eating. The heat also kills the natural enzymes in the foods that help with digestion. (Conventional ovens aren't as damaging to food because they heat more evenly; microwave ovens tend to overheat the food in certain hot spots.)

The Importance of Exercise: Putting Your Energy to Use

Carnitine not only promotes the production of energy at the cellular level, it also promotes the kind of energy that will make you feel like exercising and putting your body to use. When carnitine reserves are low, your body drags and it can be difficult to muster the energy needed to make it through a workout. When your body has access to a sufficient supply of carnitine, you will have enough drive to zip through your workout without feeling depleted.

Interestingly, exercise itself will help your body generate more energy. Exercise improves cardiovascular fitness, lowers blood pressure and cholesterol levels, improves muscle tone, strengthens the bones, and makes the joints more flexible. It improves circulation to the brain, encourages the release of soothing hormones, and helps you look and feel your best. The combination of carnitine supplementation and regular exercise provides the support your body needs to generate all the energy required to make it through a hectic day without feeling wiped out.

You don't have to spend hours in a gym to enjoy the benefits of exercise. Recent studies have shown that as little as 30 minutes a day of light physical activity will reduce your risk of disease by lowering blood pressure and cholesterol. That's physical activity, not hard-core, drip-with-sweat exercise. The time you spend strolling the neighborhood, walking the dog, climbing the stairs, and mowing the lawn counts toward the 30-minute goal. Other studies have shown that you don't even have to do your 30 minutes of activity all at once, as long as you total a half hour during the course of the day.

If you haven't worked out in a while, don't expect to overcome decades of inactivity in a couple of weeks. It took a long time to get out of shape, and it will take some time to get back in shape, so be patient. You'll start to feel the physical and psychological benefits of exercise in a few weeks, and your fitness level will continue to improve over the following months. Studies have shown that 1 year of regular exercise can return the body to a fitness level of 10 years earlier.

To get in shape, you will have to make a commitment to regular exercise; sporadic exercise won't bring the rewards of fitness. Your body will adapt to the physical demands you place on it, and it will do so without injury or discomfort, if you exercise sensibly. If you're not used to lifting anything heavier than a 10-pound bag of groceries, it will be difficult to lift a 20-pound barbell. But if you push yourself gradually, your body will adjust: Your muscles will become stronger, and your heart and lungs will begin to work more efficiently.

You can strengthen your muscles in one of three ways: by increasing the intensity of exercise (the amount of weight you lift or the speed you run), the duration of exercise (the length of time you work out), or the frequency of exercise (the number of workouts per week). As a rule of thumb, limit your overload to no more than 10 percent per week to allow your body to adjust to your fitness program gradually.

Once you start exercising, keep at it. Consistency counts. If you miss a few days of exercise, don't feel guilty and throw in the towel. Instead, just get back to it, but don't try to make up for lost time by increasing the intensity of your workout. In fact, if you skip exercise for one week, cut back on the intensity of your workout and gradually build up again.

The Benefits of Exercise

Undoubtedly you know that you should exercise, but you may not fully appreciate how important exercise can be to your overall health. Exercise can improve your physical and emotional health, reduce your risk of serious illness, and make you look years younger than your chronological age. Studies have shown that moderate exercise strengthens the body's defenses against disease; after a workout the number and aggressiveness of the white blood cells increase by 50 to 300 percent. In addition, exercise can:

- Reduce your risk of developing certain cancers, cardiovascular disease, colds and upper respiratory tract infections, diabetes (non–insulin dependent), high blood pressure, obesity, osteoarthritis, osteoporosis, and stroke
- Relieve anxiety, constipation, depression, low-back pain, and stress
- Improve your cholesterol levels; flexibility; immune system; mental alertness and reaction time; mood; muscle strength; self-esteem; sexual desire, performance, and satisfaction; short-term memory; sleep; state of relaxation; vision; and overall quality of life.

Exercise Caution

Always check with your doctor before starting an exercise program, particularly if any
of the following apply to you:

- You haven't had a medical checkup in
  more than two years.
- You're over 35.
- You're more than 30 pounds overweight.
- You have high blood pressure.
- You have high cholesterol.
- You've had a heart attack, rapid heart pal-
  pitations, or chest pain after exercise.
- You're taking or have taken heart medi-
  cation.
- Your doctor has told you that you have
  angina pectoris, fibrillation or tachycar-
  dia, an abnormal electrocardiogram (EKG),
  a heart murmur, rheumatic heart disease,
  or other heart problems.
- You smoke cigarettes.
- You have a blood relative who died of a
  heart attack before age 60.
- You have diabetes.
- You have asthma, emphysema, or any
  other lung condition.
- You get out of breath easily.
- You have arthritis or rheumatism.
- You lead a sedentary life.

The Importance of Rest: Rejuvenating Your Body with Sleep

Sleep is critical to energy production and overall health. You need a good night's sleep—for most people that means seven to nine hours of deep, uninterrupted sleep—every night in order for your immune system to work properly and for your body to work its best. Many of the people who complain of fatigue, an inability to focus, general malaise, and mild mood disorders are the same people who shortchange themselves of an appropriate amount of shut-eye.

Some people create anxiety about sleep by looking at sleep as wasted time. In truth, during periods of rest your body is rebuilding and restoring its energy system. A well-rested body is far more effective than a tired body at meeting the challenges of the day ahead. Of course, carnitine can provide the raw materials for cell metabolism and the generation of energy, but there is more to optimal health than generating energy. You also need to give your system an opportunity to rest and repair itself if you want to experience optimal health.

To promote a good night's sleep, keep the following tips in mind:

- Make a special effort to get one or two hours of extra sleep for several nights in a row. If you feel less cranky, more focused, and generally better about the day, then you should take this demonstration as a clear sign that your overall health would be improved by granting yourself several hours of extra sleep.

- If you have trouble falling asleep at night, be sure to clear your bedroom of sources of stress, especially work papers and projects that demand your attention. Try to keep your bedroom an inviting and soothing environment.

- Make sure your bedroom is dark, quiet, and well ventilated.

- Don't nap during the day, no matter how tired you feel.

- Don't fall asleep in front of the TV, including the TV in the bedroom, if you have one. Your brain must process the light and noise of the program, which cuts down on the quality of your sleep.

- Avoid eating big meals before bed. Likewise, avoid caffeine for at least three hours before bed if you have trouble falling asleep. In addition, avoid foods that can be stimulating. Foods that contain tyramines cause the brain to release norepinephrine, a stimulant. In the evening before bed, pass on tyramine-rich foods, including sugar, cheese, chocolate, sauerkraut, wine, bacon, ham, sausage, eggplant, potatoes, spinach, and tomatoes.

- Don't exercise too close to bedtime. Working out in the evening (two hours before bedtime) may help you fall asleep easily, but it can cause some people to sleep fitfully and to wake up during the night. If your exercise habits don't seem to affect your sleep, don't change them; but if you think evening or late-night exercise may compromise your sleep, try switching your exercise time to morning or midday.

- Review the prescription and nonprescription medications you are taking to find out if any could be contributing to your feelings of sleeplessness. Pain relievers, cold remedies, appetite suppressants, and decongestants as well as medications used in the treatment of asthma, hypertension, heart disease, and thyroid problems can interfere with a good night's sleep.

- Make a point to wake up at the same time each day, even if you still feel sleepy. You want to help your body establish regular sleep cycles.

- Avoid alcohol before bed. That before-bed nightcap might make you feel sleepy at first, but it will make you more likely to awaken during the night.

- If you're in the throes of a bout of insomnia and you simply can't fall sleep, do your best to stay calm and not worry about the lack of sleep. Try meditation or relaxation techniques to calm and center yourself. Keep in mind that it is relatively easy for the body to "catch up" on sleep. A single night of full sleep—one in which you sleep until you naturally awaken—will allow you to regain about 90 percent of the mental sharpness you lost due to sleep deprivation. Add a second full night, and you should be as sharp as ever.

- If you tend to awaken in the middle of the night, your blood-sugar levels may be falling too low. To avoid the problem, try having a high-carbohydrate snack before bed. Milk, whole-grain crackers, peanut butter, and bananas are particularly good choices because they contain the sleep-inducing chemical tryptophan, in addition to being good sources of carbohydrates, which can help your body maintain a moderate blood-sugar level into the night.

- In severe cases of insomnia, your doctor may prescribe drugs to promote sleep. Each year 4 to 6 million American have prescriptions filled for sleep-inducing sedatives. Never take sleeping pills for more than two weeks; while they help bring on sleep, they actually interfere with deep sleep. In addition, they can cause a "hangover" effect, in which fatigue persists during the waking hours.

The information in this chapter should get you on the way toward using carnitine in your strategy of health. Of course, you may have additional questions or concerns about the use of carnitine and other supplements. The following chapter should help clarify any remaining concerns you might have about the safe and effective use of carnitine.

TEN

Questions and Answers About Carnitine

THIS CHAPTER COVERS SOME OF THE COMMON questions or concerns about using carnitine as part of an overall approach to wellness.

Q: How long do I need to take carnitine before I will start to feel its effects?

A: Most people begin to feel the energizing effects of carnitine within a week or two of the time they start taking it. For others, however, it may take as long as a month to feel the first signs that carnitine is working its magic. If you do not experience a change in your health within four weeks, you may not be taking enough. Increase the dose by 500 milligrams a day.

If you are taking carnitine to improve your sports performance or athletic endurance, take it for at least 6 weeks before increasing your dosage. If you are taking carnitine to improve your cardiovascular health, take the supplement for 12 weeks, then work with your doctor to reassess your state of cardiovascular fitness.

In most people, the first indications of improved health include better physical stamina, sharper mental focus, or improved overall mood. Everybody has a different metabolism and will respond to carnitine (or any other nutritional supplement) at a different rate. Be patient; the benefits will be well worth the wait.

Q: Once I experience the benefits of taking carnitine, how long should I continue to take it?

A: All the evidence indicates that you can take carnitine for months or even years without experiencing any harmful side effects. In fact, a number of clinical studies on carnitine have lasted more than one year at a dose of as much as 2 grams per day. If you plan to take carnitine for a year or more, then discuss the matter with your healthcare provider.

Q: I am a strict vegetarian. I know that carnitine is found in meat and other animal products. Is carnitine an appropriate supplement for a vegetarian?

A: Because vegetarians consume little dietary carnitine, they definitely can benefit from carnitine supplements. Rest assured, carnitine itself is synthetically produced and does not contain any animal products. (If it were, it would be unaffordably expensive.) Your only potential pitfalls involve the binders and flow agents (which sometimes are made from animal products) and the gelatin capsules (which may be made from animal gelatin). If you have any questions about how a particular product is made, contact the manufacturer listed on the product label and ask for details about the manufacturing practices. Carnitine is a safe and beneficial nutritional supplement for vegetarians and carnivores alike.

Q: How much carnitine can I take without experiencing negative side effects?

A: Many people take as much as 4 grams (4,000 mg) of carnitine every day without having any unpleasant side effects. People participating in some clinical studies have consumed a whopping 15 grams (15,000 mg) of carnitine per day, with only the occasional complaint of periodic diarrhea and difficulty falling asleep.

While high doses of carnitine may not harm you, they may not help you either. Excess carnitine is excreted by the body; ultra-high doses of carnitine may not cause physical harm, but they certainly can cause financial harm.

Q: It seems that my energy level has

dropped significantly since I turned 40. Should I begin to take carnitine?

A: You should if you want to experience your youthful energy again. Many people begin taking carnitine supplements around age 40 to keep the mitochondria in their cells working at optimal levels.

Q: I have been taking carnitine three times a day, including a final dose with dinner. I sometimes find it difficult to fall asleep. Could the carnitine be disturbing my sleep?

A: Since carnitine is an energizing supplement, it can be too stimulating for some people to take later in the day. Try dividing your doses between your morning and midday meal; you should be able to enjoy a good night's sleep. If you continue to have problems, cut back on your dose by 500 milligrams a day. Also avoid caffeine, which is a stimulant as well.

Q: How can I know whether the health benefits I am experiencing are due to carnitine or some other factor?

A: One way of determining whether a supplement is responsible for health benefits is to go off them for a period of assessment. This is a "washout" period, during which time the carnitine (or any other supplement) is washed out of the body. After taking carnitine for 8 to 10 weeks, you might consider discontinuing use to see how you feel. If you believe you felt better when taking the carnitine, consider taking it again after a 4-week break.

Q: When I have taken supplements in the past, I have sometimes forgotten to take a dose. Am I at any risk if I fail to take my carnitine on a regular basis?

A: To maximize its effectiveness, you need to take your carnitine on a regular basis. If you are taking any medication for your heart, you should make carnitine a regular part of your medicine-taking routine since it can alter the amount of medication you need. Again, be sure to discuss the use of carnitine with your doctor, particularly if you have any cardiovascular problems.

Q: Where should I buy carnitine and other nutritional supplements?

A: Carnitine and other supplements are sold at health food stores, supermarkets, pharmacies, and on the Internet. One source is no better than another; you should buy supplements wherever you find them most economical and convenient to buy.

Q: Are there any special features I should look for on the product label?

A: Yes. A high-quality product should come in a tamperproof package with both an inside and outside seal. Look for products that state on the label that they are laboratory-tested and guaranteed. Before buying carnitine or any other nutritional supplement, check the product's expiration date; out-of-date supplements lose their effectiveness. Reputable manufacturers also provide a quality control number on the package, which allows the quick removal of a product from store shelves on the rare occasion that something is wrong with a given batch.

Q: Is it safe to take other vitamins or supplements while taking carnitine? Should I take a multivitamin?

A: It is perfectly safe to take carnitine along with other supplements. Multivitamins provide relatively low doses of a wide range of vitamins and minerals. They offer some assurance that your body is taking in minimal levels of key nutrients. Supplements should not be viewed as a substitute for a well-balanced diet. Healthful foods offer the best source of nutrition, but you may benefit through the strategic use of nutrients such as carnitine.

Q: Can I overdose on carnitine or CoQ10?

A: Carnitine and CoQ10 appear to be nontoxic, even at high doses. However, there is no reason to take excessively high doses. If some is good, more is not necessarily better. Your body can put only so much carnitine and CoQ10 to use at a given time; the excess is simply excreted in the urine. Taking carnitine in excess of 4 grams or so can lead to diarrhea or restlessness, but it does not appear to cause any significant health problems.

Q: Does the U.S. Food and Drug Administration approve carnitine supplements?

A: It depends on whether you buy a prescription or an over-the-counter product. Unlike most other nutritional supplements, carnitine is sold in both prescription and nonprescription forms. The prescription version must pass muster with the FDA; the over-the-counter version is unregulated by the federal government.

For the most part, the FDA does not concern itself with the production of nutritional supplements. While the FDA monitors the quality controls at drug manufacturing facilities, it does not pay much attention to the manufacturing standards of nutritional supplements.

That's not to say supplement manufacturers play fast and loose with quality controls. In fact, many supplement makers have established their own production and quality control standards, some of which are as strict as the standards imposed on pharmaceutical companies. Some supplement manufacturers test every batch of their products, looking for consistency in the amounts of active ingredients.

If you want to know about how a specific manufacturer produces its carnitine products, contact the company and ask about the testing and quality control procedures. The name and phone number of the manufacturer should be listed right on the product label. Keep in mind that manufacturers that put a lot of energy into quality control will be delighted to give you an earful about the safety and efficacy of their products.

Q: Is there any way to get my insurance company to pay for my carnitine?

A: It depends on whether your physician will write a prescription for carnitine and whether your insurance company will pay to have the prescription filled. For most people, supplements, including carnitine, must be paid for out of pocket.

Q: I am undergoing treatment for cancer. Is it safe to use carnitine and CoQ10 during my recovery?

A: It depends on the type of cancer treatment you are undergoing. Carnitine and CoQ10 have been shown to improve the effectiveness of chemotherapy and to minimize the unpleasant side effects of these treatments. CoQ10 has been found to interfere with the effectiveness of radiation treatment, however. Before using CoQ10 or carnitine during treatment, discuss the matter with your oncologist or healthcare professional.

Organizations of Interest

**American Association of Naturopathic
  Physicians**
601 Valley Street
Suite 105
Seattle, WA 98109
(206) 298-0125
www.naturopathic.org

This organization can provide referrals to naturopathic physicians who are members. In addition, the group offers brochures and background information on naturopathic medicine.

Designs for Health Institute
1750 30th Street, #319
Boulder, CO 80301
(303) 415-0229
www.dfhi.com

This group helps you find a nutritionist to aid you in developing a customized eating plan to meet your specific nutritional needs.

Institute for Traditional Medicine
2017 Southeast Hawthorne
Portland, OR 97214
(508) 233-4907
www.itmonline.org

This nonprofit institute provides educational materials and conducts research on natural healing for health professionals and interested consumers.

National College of Naturopathic Medicine
11231 S.E. Market Street
Portland, OR 97216
(503) 255-4860
www.ncnm.edu

This group can provide a referral to a naturopath or a medical doctor who specializes in natural treatments.

NUTRITION

If you have special nutritional needs or want help in designing a nutrition regimen to help manage your specific health needs, you may want to consult a nutrition counselor. For information on finding a qualified nutritionist, contact:

**American Association of Nutritional
   Consultants**
880 Canarios Court, Suite 210
Chula Vista, CA 91910-7810
(619) 482-8533

American Academy of Nutrition
3408 Sausalito Drive
Corona Del Mar, CA 92625
(800) 290-4226
www.nutritioneducation.com

American College of Nutrition
722 Robert E. Lee Drive
Wilmington, NC 28412
(919) 452-1222
www.am-coll-nutr.org

Consumer Nutrition Hotline
(Sponsored by The American Dietetic Association)
(800) 366-1655
www.eatright.org

The hotline staff can answer questions and
provide free referrals to registered dieti-
tians in your area.

Publications on nutrition are available (some for
a fee) from:

American Council on Science and Health
1995 Broadway, 16th Floor
New York, NY 10023-5860
(212) 362-7044
www.acsh.org

American Institute of Nutrition
9650 Rockville Pike, Suite L4500
Bethesda, MD 20814-3990
(301) 530-7050

The Nutrition Action Health Letter
Center for Science in the Public Interest
1875 Connecticut Avenue, NW, Suite 300
Washington, DC 20009-5728
(202) 332-9111
www. cspinet. org

Society for Nutrition Education
2001 Killebrew Drive, Suite 340
Minneapolis, MN 55425-1882
(612) 854-0035

Vegetarian Resource Group
P.O. Box 1463
Baltimore, MD 21203
(410) 366-8343
www.vrg.org

Websites of Interest

The following is a partial list of valuable medical and health sites on the Internet:

The Alternative Medicine Homepage
www.pitt.edu/~cbw/altm.html

Ask Dr. Weil
www.drweil.com

Ask the Dietitian
www.hoptechno.com/rdindex.htm

General Complementary Medicine References
www.forthrt.com/~chronicl/archiv.htm

Harvard Health Publications
www.health.harvard.edu

HealthGate
www.healthgate.com

HealthWorldOnline
www.healthy.net

Institute for Traditional Medicine
www.itmonline.org

MedWeb
www.medweb.com

Articles of Interest

Ames, B. N. "Micronutrients Prevent Cancer and Delay Aging." *Toxicology Letters* 102–03, (December 28, 1998): 5–18.

Ames, B. N., M. K. Shigenaga, and T. M. Hagen. "Oxidants, Antioxidants, and the Degenerative Diseases of Aging." *Proceedings of the National Academy of Sciences of the United States of America* 90 (1993): 7915–22.

Anand I., Y. Chandrashekhan, et al. "Acute and Chronic Effects of Propionyl-L-Carnitine on the Hemodynamics, Exercise Capacity, and Hormones in Patients with Congestive Heart Failure." *Cardiovascular Drugs Therapy* 12 (3) (July 1998): 291–99.

Arenas, J., J. C. Rubio, et al. "Biological Roles of L-Carnitine in Perinatal Metabolism." *Early Human Development* 53 Suppl. (December 1998): S43–S50.

Arsenian, M. A. "Carnitine and Its Derivatives in Cardiovascular Disease." *Progress in Cardiovascular Diseases* 40 (3) (1997): 265–86.

Atar, D., M. Spiess, A. Mandinova, et al. "Carnitine—From Cellular Mechanisms to Potential Clinical Applications in Heart Disease." *European Journal of Clinical Investigation* 27 (1997): 973–76.

Baggio, E., R. Gandini, A. C. Plancher, et al. "Italian Multicenter Study on the Safety and Efficacy of Coenzyme Q10 as Adjunctive Therapy in Heart Failure." *Molecular Aspects of Medicine* 15 Suppl. (1994): S287–S294.

Bertelli, A., L. Giovannini, et al. "Protective Synergic Effect of Coenzyme Q10 and Carnitine on Hyperbaric Oxygen Toxicity." *International Journal of Tissue Reactions* 12 (3) (1990): 193–96.

Brass, E. P., and W. R. Hiatt. "The Role of Carnitine and Carnitine Supplementation During Exercise in Man and in Individuals with Special Needs." *Journal of the American College of Nutrition*, 17 (3) (1998): 207–15.

Brass, E. P., and W. R. Hiatt. "Minireview: Carnitine Metabolism During Exercise." *Life Sciences* 54 (19) (1994): 1383–93.

Cacciatore, L., R. Cerio, M. Ciarimboli, et al. "The Therapeutic Effect of L-Carnitine in Patients with Exercise Induced Stable Angina: A Controlled Study." *Drugs Under Experimental and Clinical Research* 17 (4) (1991): 225–35.

Campoy, C., R. Bayes, et al. "Evaluation of Carnitine Nutritional Status in Full-Term Newborn Infants." *Early Human Development* 53 Suppl. (December 1998): S139–S164.

Capurso, A., F. Resta, M. Colacicco, et al. "Effect of L-Carnitine on Elevated Lipoprotein (a) Levels." *Current Therapeutic Research* 56 (12) (1995): 1247–53.

DeVivo, D. C., T. P. Bohan, et al. "L-Carnitine Supplementation in Childhood Epilepsy: Current Perspectives." *Epilepsia* 39 (11) (November 1998): 1216–25.

Ellaway, C., K. Williams, et al. "Rett Syndrome: Randomized Controlled Trial of L-Carnitine." *Journal of Child Neurology* 14 (3) (March 1999): 162–67.

Freeman, L. M. "Interventional Nutrition for Cardiac Disease." *Clinical Techniques in Small Animal Practice* 13 (4) (November 1998): 232–37.

Gabauer, I., I. Pechan, Fischer, et al. "Cardioprotection of L-Carnitine in Patients During Coronary Surgery." *Journal of Molecular and Cellular Cardiology* 29 (5) (1997): S12.

Gunal, A. I., et al. "The Effect of L-Carnitine on Insulin Resistance in Hemodialysed Patients with Chronic Renal Failure." *Journal of Nephrology* 12 (1) (January-February 1999): 38–40.

Hagen, T. M., R. T. Ingersoll, et al. "Acetyl-L-Carnitine Fed to Old Rats Partially Restores Mitochondrial Function and Ambulatory Activity." *Proceedings of the National Academy of Sciences* 95 (16) (August 4, 1988): 9562–66.

Hagen, T. M., C. M. Wehr, and B. N. Ames. "Mitochondrial Decay in Aging. Reversal through Supplementation of Acetyl-L-Carnitine." *Annals of the New York Academy of Sciences* 854 (November 20, 1998): 214–23.

Kamikawa, T., A. Kobayashi, et al. "Effects of Coenzyme Q10 on Exercise Tolerance in

Chronic Stable Angina Pectoris." *American Journal of Cardiology* 56 (1985): 247–51.

Keller, V. A., B. Toporoff, et al. "Carnitine Supplementation Improves Myocardial Function in Hearts from Ischemic Diabetic and Euglycemic Rats." *Annals of Thoracic Surgery,* 66 (5) (November 1998): 1600–3.

Kelly, G. S. "L-Carnitine: Therapeutic Applications of a Conditionally-Essential Amino Acid." *Alternative Medicine Review* 3 (5) (October 1998): 345–60.

Krahenbuhl, S., B. Willer, et al. "Carnitine homeostasis in Patients with Rheumatoid Arthritis." *Clinica Chimica Acta: International Journal of Clinical Chemistry* 279 (102) (January 1999): 35–45.

Kuratsune, H., K. Yamaguti, et al. "Low Levels of Serum Acylcarnitine in Chronic Fatigue Syndrome and Chronic Hepatitis Type C, But Not Seen in Other Diseases." *International Journal of Molecular Medicine* 2 (1) (July 1998) 51–56.

Marconi, C., G. Sassi, et al. "Effects of L-Carnitine Loading on the Aerobic and Anaerobic Performance of Endurance Athletes." *European Journal of Applied Physiology* 54 (1985): 131–35.

Mecocci, P., U. MacGarvey, et al. "Oxidative Damage to Mitochondrial DNA Shows Marked Age-Dependent Increase in Human

Brain." *Annals of Neurology* 34 (4) (1993): 609–16.

Mingrone, G., A. V. Greco, et al. "L-Carnitine Improves Glucose Disposal in Type 2 Diabetic Patients." *Journal of the American College of Nutrition* 18 (1) (February 1999): 77–82.

Narin, F., N. Narin, et al. "Carnitine Levels in Patients with Chronic Rheumatic Heart Disease." *Clinical Biochemistry* 30 (8) (December 1997): 643–65.

Pastoris, O., M. Dossena, et al. "Effect of L-Carnitine on Myocardial Metabolism: Results of a Balanced, Placebo-Controlled, Double-Blind Study in Patients Undergoing Open Heart Surgery." *International Journal of Clinical Pharmacology Research* 37 (2) (February 1998): 115–22.

Paulson, D. J. "Carnitine Deficiency-Induced Cardiomyopathy." *Molecular and Cellular Biochemistry* 180 (1–2) (March 1998): 33–41.

Penn, D., L. Zhang, et al. "Carnitine Deprivation Adversely Affects Cardiac Performance in the Lipopolysaccharide- and Hypoxia/ Reoxygenation-Stressed Piglet Heart." *Shock* 11 (2) (February 1999): 120–26.

Pettegrew, J. W., W. E. Klunck, et al. "Clinical and Neurochemical Effects of Acetyl-L-Carnitine in Alzheimer's Disease." *Neurobiology of Aging* 16 (1) (1995): 1–4.

Plioplys, A., and S. Plioplys. "Amantadine and

L-Carnitine Treatment of Chronic Fatigue Syndrome." *Neuropsychobiology* 35 (1997): 16–23.

Sakurauchi, Y., Y. Matsumoto, et al. "Effects of L-Carnitine Supplementation on Muscular Symptoms in Hemodialyzed Patients." *American Journal of Kidney Disease* 32 (2) (August 1998): 258–64.

Shannon, D. W., and G. S. Wolfe, "Carnitine Deficiency: A Missed Diagnosis." *Journal of Care Management* 3 (3) (1997): 12–24.

Shigenaga, M. K., T. M. Hagen, and B. N. Ames. "Oxidative Damage and Mitochondrial Decay in Aging." *Proceedings of the National Academy of Sciences* 91 (1994): 10771–78.

Sloan, R. S., B. Kastan, et al. "Quality of Life During and Between Hemodialysis Treatments: Role of L-Carnitine Supplemenation." *American Journal of Kidney Disease* 32 (2) (August 1998): 265–72.

Swartz, I., et al. "The Effect of L-Carnitine Supplementation on Plasma Carnitine Levels and Various Performance Parameters of Male Marathon Athletes." *Nutrition Research* 17 (1997): 405–14.

Virmani, M. A., R. Biselli, et al. "Protective Actions of L-Carnitine and Acetyl-L-Carnitine on the Neurotoxicity Evoked by Mitochondrial Uncoupling or Inhibitors." *Pharmacological Research* 32 (6) (1995): 383–89.

Watanabe, S., R. Ajisake, et al. "Effects of L- and DL- Carnitine on Patients with Impaired Exercise Tolerance." *Japanese Heart Journal* 36 (3) (1995): 319–31.